Drugless Medicine

by the same author

Stress Disease: the Growing Plague
Hypnotism: Its Power and Practice

Peter Blythe

Drugless Medicine

Arthur Barker Limited   London
A subsidiary of Weidenfeld (Publishers) Limited

Arthur Barker Limited 11 St John's Hill London SW11

ISBN 0 213 16471 X
Printed in Great Britain by
Bristol Typesetting Co Ltd
Barton Manor St Philips
Bristol

This book is dedicated to
my father, Henry Blythe

Contents

Preface

'It is about time that someone wrote a book about drugless medicines that can be used instead of the piles of pills that doctors are always prescribing,' is how one of my friends encouraged me when he learned of my plans to write this book. However, as it began to take shape the same person, and others who had originally been enthusiastic about the project, began to change their minds. On more than one occasion I was accused of attacking the medical profession, and was forcibly told that what I was writing would encourage the growth of *quackery*.

I cannot deny that in the course of researching the contents of this work I became highly critical of certain aspects of organized orthodox medicine, and I found it particularly frightening when I was confronted with examples where the orthodox medical hierarchy took upon itself the role of Dictator; deciding without clinical trial and experiment that certain therapies were useless although there was ample evidence to show they may be efficacious.

Yet, at the same time, many orthodox medical practitioners went up in my esteem.

When I talked to these doctors they were ready to admit that alternative medical practitioners, the so-called 'Fringe-medicine Men', had a lot to offer patients, and they regretted that they were prevented by a strict Code of Ethics forced upon them from sending individual patients to them when they felt they would benefit.

The dilemma those physicians found themselves in is to some degree my own dilemma.

That alternative medicine has a role to play in modern medicine became obvious to me, and in the following pages I have tried to present the evidence which led me to that conclusion, but this conclusion does not mean that I think orthodox medicine should be discarded as being an *enemy* to health as some Nature Cure practitioners postulate. Instead I feel the time has come – and perhaps it has long passed – when all branches of medicine should get together in a type of therapeutic 'ecumenical council' to establish how they can work together with equal parity, and in harmony, for the benefit of those people who have fallen victim to disease.

Peter Blythe
4 Stanley Place
Chester

July, 1973

Acknowledgements

I wish to acknowledge the help given to me by Mr John Hyde of the National Institute of Medical Herbalists, Mr D. Emlyn Roberts, and many other members of the Institute. J. Hewlett-Parsons of the General Council and Register of Consultant Herbalists, Miss June Johns, Mr Sidney Rose-Neil of Tyringham Naturopathic Clinic, Mr Terry Ryan, Mrs Valerie Gilmore, Mr Stan Duncombe, Dr John R. Denton, DC, of the Anglo-European College of Chiropractic, Mr Ken Woodward of the Northern Institute of Massage, Mr Deryk Kemp and many others.

In acknowledging the assistance given to me I must make it clear that what I have written need not entirely meet with the approval of those who have given me information, because I felt I had to be free to take what I thought to be important and to give my own interpretations of the material. I hope this is acceptable to them.

Nor would this book have been possible without the many clients I have seen over the years.

I

Where Has My Doctor Gone?

'My doctor isn't really interested in me. He never listens when I try to tell him what is wrong; he is far too busy writing out a prescription for me.' This is how more and more people are expressing their dissatisfaction with the treatment they are receiving from their General Practitioner.

Naturally many members of the medical profession deny that this type of accusation could be levelled against them, but during the course of a lecture I gave recently dealing with the importance of verbal communication I asked the members of the large audience how many of them felt they had experienced this type of rejection from their medical practitioner, and only two of them could state without any hesitation that their doctor did *not* treat them in this offhand manner.

Yet, is this criticism fair? Is the friendly General Practitioner, the true family doctor, still in practice or has he fallen victim to the impersonalism which appears to have pervaded every aspect of life in our industrialized society?

One way to find part of the answer to both of these questions can be done by conducting a simple experiment which entails, the next time you are ill, trying to contact your own doctor during a weekend. Unless the particular doctor happens to be on rota duty that weekend and you are lucky, the chances are your telephone call will be automatically switched through to another practitioner who has no knowledge of your, the patient's, case history, or what treatment has previously been prescribed.

And it is not only patients who are becoming more and more alarmed at the depersonalization of the doctor-patient relationship, as a number of physicians have also voiced their concern at the breach which obviously exists.

Dr Hertzel Creditor, writing in the medical weekly *Pulse* under the title 'Preparing for Practice',[1] described how older doctors could remember the past, and how 'General Practice was conducted then . . . with an understanding of humanity, a decency that is not easily discerned today.' Later in the same article she added that the General Practitioner 'must be interested in other people's illnesses and their response to them, otherwise he should be sent off to work in a laboratory. He needs to be involved with his patients, involved with illness as well as with "medicine".'

In a further article which Dr Creditor wrote in *Pulse* a little less than a month later, entitled 'Friend and Counsellor Image is Vanishing Fast',[2] she said that the GP should come out into the open and tell his patients if he intends to forget all about being the family friend and counsellor so that the patient will know exactly where he or she stands with regard to their one-time close relationship. She also drew her colleagues' attention to the new and frustrating habit of shutting off the telephone at weekends, or having an automatic answering machine at the other end, which she says is equivalent to telling the patient, ' "I don't like you. I don't want you. I don't wish to speak to you." ' And when Dr Creditor spoke on the same theme at a medical symposium she wrote that she was '. . . howled down by a pack of braying GPs!'

While very few people who have experienced the type of rejection Dr Creditor mentions would disagree with her assessment, the doctor did not take her argument far enough according to some patients and doctors, as they consider the barriers which have been erected potentially dangerous.

This was highlighted recently when a middle-aged gentleman had a heart attack early one Friday evening. The man's wife, in a state of alarm, telephoned their own doctor, but the call was intercepted and redirected to another doctor's number. The wife explained to the lady who answered the call that she thought her husband had had a coronary, and requested that the doctor visit her husband immediately. 'I am afraid he is out at the moment on another call,' was the answer she got, together with the assurance that when the doctor returned the message would be given to him for immediate attention.

Half an hour later there was no sign of the doctor, but fortunately the son of the couple arrived, and after taking one look at his father telephoned the emergency service and was put through to the ambulance service, with the result that he was taken straight into hospital.

Upon arrival the patient was taken to the intensive care unit as his condition was critical, and the son was informed that if admission had been delayed any longer the heart attack could have proved fatal.

Having assured himself that his father was receiving the best possible care the son returned home to be told by his mother that although nearly two hours had elapsed since the doctor had been telephoned he still had not arrived to examine the patient. In other words the father could well have died in the interim.

'Why hadn't the doctor got a radio receiver in his car so that he could have been notified of the emergency?' was the reaction of a friend who heard this near tragic story. One answer put forward is that they are too expensive for most GPs in Britain, but when countered with 'Isn't the saving of a life worth the monetary outlay?' there is no realistic argument proferred. Another answer is that there could be a breakdown in the confidential relationship between the doctor and the patient as such telephone calls can be overheard or intercepted. This too lacks any degree of realistic validity, as an identical leak could occur in those instances when the patient telephones the doctor at his surgery.

However, returning to the examination of the vanishing family doctor, an Essex GP, writing under the pseudonym of Dr Jane Finlay, said, 'patients suffer because relationships with GPs are too distant,' and that doctors 'are taught to find a disease they can treat more or less successfully,' and if there is no physical disease obviously present the patient may simply be classified as 'neurotic'. If the prevailing symptoms are mild the patient will get some form of symptomatic treatment, whereas if they are severe he or she will be shunted off to see a psychiatrist which the Essex doctor sees as 'a form of rejection practised by specialists in physical diseases. Rarely is the doctor taught to see the patient as a whole person in the setting of his family, his work and his friends.'[3]

What this doctor had to contribute to the subject raises two other important aspects which cannot be overlooked, and therefore I will attempt to deal with each of them separately.

First of all she has put her finger on the pulse of another common complaint by patients: 'They are not interested in finding out why I am ill, all they are interested in is getting me out of the surgery as quickly as possible.'

A physician I met more or less admitted this happened in most GPs' surgeries, and that he and his partners had worked out a schedule based on the average number of patients waiting to see them, which meant they had approximately two and a half minutes to devote to each person. He assured me that, due solely to the time factor, he had to treat the presenting symptom rather than try to find out why the patient had it. This mechanistic approach to general medical practice reminds me of a film I recently saw on British television called, 'Say Goodbye Maggie Cole', starring Miss Susan Hayward, where a young girl dying of leukaemia complained about her doctor's attitude towards her illness by crying out, 'I have a disease, but *I* am not a disease'. It was a heart-rending plea, echoed by many, to be treated as an individual who was sick, rather than as a specimen of a sick individual.

A more typical example of this symptomatological approach came to light in my own practice as a psychotherapist when a middle-aged gentleman came to see me suffering from insomnia which had persisted for more than a year. He was extremely disgruntled by the medical treatment he had received because, according to him, all his own doctor did was to prescribe sleeping pills, which had been unsuccessful as he still woke up in the early hours of the morning, and then stayed awake until it was time for him to get up. When he arose for the day he felt he had no energy; his life had become meaningless, and everything he did was an arduous chore.

When he finally complained to his GP that the pills were not having the desired effect, they were simply changed for another pill. When he asked, 'How long will I have to go on like this? And when you do find the right pill to put me to sleep, does it mean I shall have to continue taking them for the remainder of my life?' the doctor made no reply, and the client said to me that he had been forced to come and see me because he had reached the conclusion that he was being treated by a hit-and-miss technique, and that the doctor was not interested in finding out why he was unable to sleep.

As I am not a registered medical practitioner in the accepted sense of the terminology, and therefore unable to prescribe drugs, a procedure which would have been valueless anyway as his need to be awake at night was obviously stronger than his desire to sleep, at our initial consultation I got the client to tell me about his past; not only about his previous illnesses, although they too were important if I was to understand his personality, but to tell me about those times when he had been under stress and his sleeping pattern had been disturbed.

Without any prompting on my part he related that, back in the 1940s his wife had been dying of an incurable disease, and that for two years he had learned to sleep intermittently, with one ear and one eye open in case she needed attention during the night, which she frequently did. For six months after her death he was unable to sleep properly, then as he recovered from his sense of personal loss he began to sleep normally again. Until 1972 he suffered no recurrence of insomnia, but then he had a coronary in the early hours of the morning and was subsequently hospitalized. And that was when the problem reappeared, and had continued to plague him ever since.

I asked him why he felt being in hospital had prevented him from sleeping, and he told me it was because someone was continually moving around the ward.

In the few minutes it took him to tell me the background to his insomnia, a most probable answer became apparent. Being awoken in the early hours of the morning by his heart attack, together with people moving around the ward in hospital, had reactivated the behavioural pattern previously learned when he had to sleep with an eye and an ear cocked in case his wife needed him.

My tentative analysis of his basic problem could have been wrong. The origin could have stemmed from his being afraid to sleep in case he had a further coronary in the middle of the night and was not awake to tell anyone of his predicament. Not being endowed with second sight or having a diagnostic crystal ball, and because I believe it is wrong for any practitioner dealing with these psychogenic problems to tell the patient or client what he thinks is wrong with him, since he should rather assist the person to reach an understanding of what lies behind the symptom, I used a type of hypnotic diagnosis I had developed, to ascertain what was the real reason.[4] In this instance my earlier conclusion proved to be correct, so immediately after the hypno-diagnostic session had been terminated I explained to him how he had 'learned' not to sleep, and how his earlier learning in the 1940s had been reactivated by his time in hospital.

To assist his comprehension I quoted a couple of examples of how, once a behavioural pattern is learned, it is very easily reactivated.

I explained how a person can learn to drive a car, and then does not drive again for many years. When he gets behind the steering wheel again he may find it strange for a few minutes, but within a very short period he begins to drive automatically as the earlier learning pattern is reactivated. In the same way, a cigarette smoker may break the smoking habit and remain a non-smoker for a considerable period, but once he has a single cigarette it isn't long before he is back into his old learned habit and smoking twenty a day.

Although I used hypnosis, and the appropriate suggestions, to restore a normal sleep pattern to this client, I am sure that if his own doctor had taken the time to listen to what the patient could have told him about the genesis of his sleep problem, and explained to him about learned behavioural patterns, he would have found the drugs he prescribed would have been effective, and before long his patient would have been able to sleep without them.

The second factor which Dr 'Jane Finlay's' article touched upon was that doctors in general practice are not taught how to deal with people, but only with diseases.

The Royal College of General Practitioners has recognized this omission in the medical training syllabus, and is currently trying to correct it by establishing Vocational Training Schemes for GPs, but these are proving to be unpopular, so that patients cannot really expect a general change in medical attitudes until doctors receive an adequate part of their training actually working in a general practice instead of becoming disease-specialists in a hospital.

Having made this slight deviation from the main theme, I would suggest that the rapid development of group medical practices throughout the British Isles has been a major contributory factor to the barrier between physician and patient. For prior to their inception the patient felt he or she had their own doctor, someone with whom there was a continuity of contact. Today, if a group comprises three or more doctors, they tend to operate on a rota system for daily surgeries, and a patient has no way of knowing which of them he will see, thereby preventing personal identification with 'my doctor'.

On the surface group practices may appear to be more efficient, but in addition to depersonalizing the doctor-patient relationship they are detrimental to the reputation of individual doctors.

Patients have the opportunity of comparing the doctors within the group and how they treat them, and quickly decide, perhaps on an emotive level and without justification, that Dr X has no idea about what he is doing, while Dr Y is a superior practitioner. Having made their value-judgements the patients proclaim their opinions, and others begin to accept their evaluation.

A more harmful feature of the group concept is that it makes the patients feel they are unimportant, nothing more nor less than faceless file-cards which can be pulled out by any doctor who happens to be taking the surgery they attend. Nor is the feeling of being relegated to mere ciphers without some validity.

In a north-western town of England a group of doctors arbitrarily decided they would not hold any evening surgeries, a decision which led to widespread private and public protest because there was no other doctor outside the group practising in the town.

Men who were working during the day but who wanted to visit the doctor had to take time away from work to do so, and not all employers were agreeable to them having temporary leave of absence. Women with small children who would normally leave them with their husbands after they got home in the evenings had difficulty in finding baby-sitters. The protests against this decision grew. People complained to their local council representatives, but the councillors were unable to prevail upon the doctors to reconsider their attitude. Thwarted at that level, people sent further complaints to the government department responsible for the National Health Service. Back came the answer that under the terms of their contracts with the Health Service doctors could not be compelled to hold evening surgeries. As the storm mounted the regional independent television station investigated the situation, and as it was intended to televize its findings the doctors in the group were invited to appear on TV to put forward their reasons for the decision. The invitation was rejected. Eventually the problem was solved when another doctor moved into the town and agreed to hold an evening surgery, although those local people who had been patients of the group practitioners and had been vocally active in complaining were informed they should seek future medical care elsewhere.

As far as that town was concerned the image of the family doctor had disappeared, to be replaced by that of the medical autocrat.

To make these matters worse, if that were possible, the appointment system has been brought into being, allegedly to assist the patient, and to prevent large numbers from spending unnecessary time in the waiting-room. According to complaints received by the Patients' Association the scheme frequently prevents patients from seeing their doctor within a reasonable period of time.

In a news item appearing in *The Daily Telegraph* on 27 March 1973, the Patients' Association stated this had become the biggest cause of complaint. Some patients found they would make an appointment, arrive on time, and then have to sit with a group of other people waiting for the doctor to arrive. The chairman of the Association, Mrs Helen Hodgson, told *The Daily Telegraph,* 'To wait for an appointment and then wait again is really disgraceful.'

And even to get an appointment is not always simple for those people who have not got a telephone in the house, or who dislike using them – and many older people fall into the latter category – and when this is the case it means making two visits to the surgery, one to make the appointment, and another to see the doctor.

There have been cases cited where a patient had to wait fourteen days for an appointment, and according to Mrs Hodgson one woman was told she would have to wait four days to see the doctor. When she made loud and long protests to the effect that she could not wait that long the doctor examined her immediately, but informed her as he handed over the prescription that she was no longer welcome on his list as a patient and had better look elsewhere.

Answering these accusations a spokesman for the Royal College of General Practitioners admitted that receptionists were deciding if a patient was sufficiently ill enough to have an immediate appointment or whether they could wait a few days, and said, 'But in such cases the practice is not properly organized or the receptionist has been wrongly advised by the doctor.'

Of course it would be totally unfair to put all the blame for what is happening solely upon the shoulders of the medical profession; patients too are partly responsible for the form of conveyor-belt medicine now becoming so prevalent. Prior to the inception of the appointment system many people saw going to the doctor as a social occasion, and waiting-rooms throughout Britain were regularly jammed full of people who made their weekly visit a ritual. This became apparent to me while I was discussing the changes taking place in general practice with a doctor and his wife.

It was the doctor's wife who told me how she had been in the dispensary next to the waiting-room when she overheard the following conversation. A habitual patient greeted another who had just arrived with the observation, 'I missed you last Tuesday.' To which the reply was, 'Yes, I was too ill to come.'

That may sound like a second-rate comedian's joke, but it was typical of a widespread, prevailing attitude, and if the doctor attempted to correct this misuse and abuse of his time by saying that the patient need not come so often, he would be told. 'We pay for the National Health Service, and you get paid by our contributions, so I shall come as often as I want to.' And the poor doctor faced with such a retort could only implore the habitual patient to think of the others who were really sick and needed his attention.

Another medical manoeuvre to combat the wasting of the doctor's time was to give a prescription for a long-term supply of medicine or pills with the instruction, 'Come back and see me when you have finished taking them.' But that led to serious complications, such as the misuse of drugs. People would pass along the remnants of their prescription to a friend who felt that he had not got the time to spare hanging around a doctor's waiting-room for an hour or so. Others would accidentally take an overdose.

When these tactics failed, the implementation of group medical practices and of the appointment system were the next logical step. However, many people believe this was not done to assist the patient, as medical spokesmen state, but was inspired by doctors feeling there was a need to put up a barrier between them and their habitual patients, and to make it more difficult for people to see them. As one doctor said, 'The underlying logic is: if it takes some effort before they, the patients, can get through to me, then only those who really need my services will take the trouble.'

If his assessment of the motivation for the 'improvements' is correct, then it has been successful. For the barrier is now well and truly erected, the tragedy being that the doctor, the friend and confidant, has disappeared behind it and can no longer be seen or trusted.

A prominent London General Practitioner, Dr John Macrae, who is a strong critic of the appointment system, expressed a different viewpoint. According to him it had been introduced to 'boost the slumping morale of the family doctor'. And his view about the poor morale was summed up when he told *The Daily*

Telegraph,[5] 'The Royal College of General Practitioners has not got the guts to fight the main issue – that family doctors should be allowed to supervise their patients' treatment in hospital.'

It could be argued that the opinions expressed above, with the exception of those of Dr Macrae, are unsupported and biased in order to bolster the conclusions I am presenting; that there is no real dissatisfaction with the present state of general medical practice, and that the innovations, group practices, health centres, appointments, etc. are working well; and that therefore there is nothing to worry about. To show that I am not presenting a partisan picture it would be pertinent to have a look at the official attitude towards the situation.

Not long ago a Chief Medical Officer at the Department of Health and Social Security announced that the available statistics showed that the single-practice doctor was ceasing to exist; but a responsible inquiry had revealed that the doctor working alone – outside a group practice – was happy to remain that way; and more important the inquiry showed that the patients of the solo doctor were anxious he should remain in that position. Yet the way in which the Chief Medical Officer presented the information about the growth of conveyor-belt medicine suggested that the demise of the single-practice doctor was beneficial to all concerned. This was soon shown not to be the case, because shortly afterwards the Department of Health and Social Security announced it was to set up a committee to investigate the deficiencies of general practice, and from the latter announcement it can be deduced that not only is there patient dissatisfaction, but the government also has grave doubts too.[6]

What has been outlined in this chapter so far has dealt with what is happening in Britain to drive a wedge between the patient and the doctor, although in the United States of America the same results have manifested themselves, but for different reasons.

As every American knows, from the President in the White House to the welfare recipient in a shack home, the cost of medical care has reached such mammoth proportions that millions of people cannot afford to consult a doctor. And the American physician is equally aware that he has priced himself away from the majority of his patients. This is evidenced in press reports of the 1963 meeting of the American Medical Association convention held in Atlantic City, New Jersey, where the delegates discussed as their major topic 'telling our story', and the then President of the AMA said, 'We must put over to the public why medicine costs so much.'

When it has been recognized that the basic barrier exists at a grass-root level in industrialized nations, as well as in others, there is another common denominator which makes the layman feel that medicine has become dehumanized, and this is the apparently indiscriminate use of medical specialists.

Everywhere, in every industry and profession, more and more specialists are emerging, and the medical profession is no exception. Again the development has a logical basis in keeping with the general pattern of technological advancement. For as all aspects of life become more intricate it would be well nigh impossible for any one man to be a master of every aspect of his profession. And this is accepted in medicine until the moment comes, and it has already come, when the patient feels that the suggestion 'I would like you to see a specialist' is merely buck-passing.

Doctors themselves may dislike this interpretation, and may see themselves as merely utilizing the specialist services available to them when they want a second opinion. It would be foolish to deny the reality of this where surgery may be necessary or in the rare cases when the presenting symptomatology is baffling. But a number of doctors have told me they are occasionally forced to seek a second opinion to satisfy a patient, while others have admitted they sometimes use this method to rid themselves of a troublesome patient who is always complaining, and has become a burden to them.

But let us take a look at the other side of the coin – at the British patient who is told it is necessary to see a specialist, and then has to wait until he receives notification of his appointment (and that alone can take anything from weeks to months dependent upon the specialist's availability). So the patient patiently waits. He arrives in good time for his appointment, then there is more waiting, because the appointments system in hospitals has been notoriously inefficient for years, even prior to the innovation of the Health Service in 1948.

There are times when the specialist wants more information before he can reach a diagnosis, and the patient then has to wait for yet another appointment. . . . If minor surgery is deemed necessary then another wait of anything from a few months to years can ensue, and the waiting can and does create psychological havoc.

Yet perhaps the worst buck-passing happens when the GP meets a case of neurosis which fails to respond to the familiar tranquillizers or anti-depressants. Instead of trying to get the patient to talk and to understand his or her background, which could be responsible for the symptoms, the GP gives the answer: 'I would like you to see a psychiatrist.' That gives rise to further problems for the already-disturbed patient.

Due to long-standing prejudice, the reaction to being asked to see a psychiatrist can be, 'Does the doctor think I am some form of nut? All I want is some help to tide me over this crisis.' And when the help is not forthcoming the doctor's prestige is lowered, and the man and the profession sink a little lower in esteem. Alternatively, the suggestion can cause even more anxiety as the patient concludes, 'The doctor must think I am really bad, otherwise he could have dealt with it.'

The first reaction can cause an antagonism which is allowed to continue festering while the patient waits for an appointment to see the psychiatrist, and the second can give rise to greater anxiety.

Across the Atlantic the 'I would like you to see a specialist' recommendation can be interpreted to mean the patient has to spend more money. As an American said to me while we were discussing this entire problem, 'The doctors have got a good racket going for them, and we are the suckers. They don't want us to get well quickly; for them it is "the slower the better", as that means they can all get a slice of the money-cake.'

What he did not know is that a famous American, Benjamin Franklin, had said much the same thing two centuries earlier: 'God heals, and the doctor takes the fee.'

All judgements of this nature may be harsh and exaggerated, but they do sum up how many people now feel about a profession they once respected.

2

Internal Pollution

Due to doctors being overworked, the lack of time they can spend with each patient, and the increasing number of new drugs continually flooding the medical market, the personality of the physician plays a decreasing role in treatment. This is how Dr Donald Gibson, chairman of the British Medical Association Council, assessed the situation in 1969 when he called upon his colleagues to make a concerted effort to reduce drug-induced – iatrogenic – illnesses.

Dr Gibson continued, 'So often the worried patient, who dares not openly ask an over-strained doctor for the examination which would give him the reassurance he needs, is given a prescription in lieu.

'We are encouraging the fear of physical disease and even treating it medicinally. We are indulging in pseudo-curative medicine when we should be fulfilling a more accurate role in the preventive phase.

'The unhappiness and positive misery we cause through this are incalculable.'[1]

The knowledge that the drugs being given out in ever increasing amounts are causing new illnesses has been known to the medical profession for a number of years, although the general public has not been alerted to the dangers it is facing.

At the BMA annual clinical meeting in 1969 Dr Henry Mathew, who is in charge of the Edinburgh Royal Infirmary regional poisoning treatment centre, said that ten per cent of all acute admissions to most hospitals throughout the country were suffering from acute drug-poisoning – and he was referring to medically prescribed pharmaceutical drugs, not to illegally obtained drugs – and he stated this was double the number of cases admitted with coronary thrombosis or diabetes.

Quoting statistics Dr Mathew showed that more than 1,000 patients a year were handled by his unit, and he predicted that if the epidemic remained unchecked the entire population of Edinburgh, some 500,000 people, would pass through his hands by the dreaded year of 1984.[2]

Two years after these two medical pundits sounded the alarm, a Dr Rebecca Rainsbury, researching into the effects of drugs upon human cellular and tissue systems at London University, again rang the warning bell regarding iatrogenic illness, and reiterated that ten per cent of patients in British hospitals were there because of drug pollution. However, the figure she gave is, according to other doctors who are equally concerned about the growing danger of internal drug pollution, very conservative, and the true figure is already much higher. This is confirmed by an American physician who recently wrote that approximately one quarter of non-surgical cases end up suffering from a serious drug reaction.

In 1971 Dr Rainsbury went to the United States of America to discuss and publicize the dangers of drug pollution, as she and her associates 'want to establish what risks we are running to ourselves and the next generation in liberally taking to the drug habit.' Included in the drugs she was worried about was the oral contraceptive pill being swallowed by millions of women daily throughout the world, because in her opinion no one knew the long-term effects the pill would have on future generations of mothers.

It is true that she was well received in the US, and after she had talked with Senator Teddy Kennedy, the Senator asked Congress to write into the Congressional Record a paper entitled and devoted to 'Internal Pollution', written by such eminent men as Sir Julian Huxley, Professor Jacques Monod, the Nobel Prize winner and director of the renowned Pasteur Institute, and Sir Rudolph Peters, Professor of Biochemistry at Cambridge University. Yet her trip was largely fruitless, with alarming results which are only now becoming more and more apparent.

Recently a group of doctors in Boston, Mass., have found that young women whose mothers had been given synthetic estrogen in the form of the drug Stilbestrol, to prevent them from having a miscarriage, are more prone to develop a certain type of cervical cancer as they reach the age of puberty than female children of those mothers who were not treated with Stilbestrol during pregnancy. The investigating medical team recommended that any young woman whose mother had been given synthetic estrogen should have regular vaginal examinations.

The disturbing part of this particular news item which came to light in 1973 is that hundreds of thousands of women have been given this drug during the past twenty-five years, and only now are the possible effects beginning to manifest themselves in the next generation of their female offspring.

And what is even more alarming is the knowledge that these cancer-prone manifestations could have been averted if, initially, the doctors who wrote out the Stilbestrol prescriptions had spent more time talking to the women patients with a history of miscarriages. For other practitioners have found that women who spontaneously abort their unborn children may have psychological reasons for the spontaneous termination; if the psychological origins can be detected, and if such women are given hypnotic relaxation and appropriate suggestions, many can be helped to carry their child through the nine months of pregnancy without resorting to drugs.

But doctors themselves are caught up in the drug-whirlpool, and they minimize the dangers by adopting the self-comforting attitude: 'Well, there are bound to be some side-effects in a small number of people.' This may be enough to reassure them as they continue writing out prescriptions for drugs, like printing presses churning out the morning newspapers, but iatrogenic illnesses are more than mere 'side-effects', as a heading in the *Medical News Tribune*[3] made quite clear: 'When Remedy is Worse than Disease'.

The medical newspaper then reported, 'Every doctor who prescribes drugs must be aware of the possibility that the remedy might be worse than the disease for which it is prescribed, warns a leading Dutch pharmacologist. These drug-induced diseases are so varied that there are indeed few pathological conditions that may not be brought about by some drug, Professor L. Meyler, Professor of Clinical Pharmacology at Groningen University, told the International Meeting of Medical Advisers to the Pharmaceutical Industry in London.'

When faced with this and similar warnings doctors have given me the typical retort: 'I am aware of the dangers, but what has to be kept in mind is that the drugs more often than not *are* effective, and therefore the risks involved are justified.'

This is incorrect, and while I fully appreciate that my quoting an isolated case can be dismissed as an exception to the rule, I recently became aware of a man who had a long history of nervous disorders and finally had a breakdown at work when he threw all the papers lying on his desk into the face of his boss, and was left with a paralyzed hand and arm. Instead of attempting to find out why he needed the paralysis, and of finding out what he would do if his hand and arm weren't paralyzed, a simple enough investigatory psychological procedure, the patient's doctor had put him on a course of treatment with a major tranquillizer, one of the phenothiazines, Largactil, which is a well-known and much-prescribed drug.

Within a short period of his taking Largactil the patient developed severe jaundice, and his liver rapidly deteriorated to the point where he was put on the hospital danger-list for fourteen days and was not expected to live. Then the doctors attending him admitted the drug was the cause of the trouble as his liver found it too difficult to process.

In this case the important question to be answered is, 'Was the risk worth it?'

There can be only one answer, a definite 'no'. The patient's psychosomatic syndrome may well have responded to a psychotherapeutic approach, as many psychotherapists would testify; and even if this were not possible, and surely it would have been preferable to find out if it were before using the drug, the prescribing of chlorpromazine – to give Largactil its correct name – was not the answer either. For back in the early 1960s a strict test was carried out with chlorpromazine which showed that, with certain people, it was little more than a placebo, a therapeutically valueless substance which is given to the patient with the suggestion that it has the power to cure.[4]

As Largactil is still being widely used, and people like the one I have written about in the preceding paragraphs are placed in the position where their entire health may be jeopardized by a chemical substance that has little real therapeutic value, more questions arise. How could this happen? Why do doctors allow it?

The blame must primarily be laid at the door of the drug makers, the pharmaceutical companies. They put a lot of money into researching each of their products before it is marketed; they make every attempt to ensure safety for the patient who will take it, but having done both of these things they have to try and recoup their financial outlay, even if it means trying to get doctors to use the drugs despite the dangers of side-effects or iatrogenic illnesses.

The way the drug industry tries to influence members of the medical profession is by extensive advertising in the numerous medical journals, and there is evidence that the industry's advertising executives are just as prone to exaggeration as their colleagues preparing advertisements for television.

An expert who looked into this brainwashing of doctors through the advertising media, Professor O. L. Wade, found that, out of forty-four drugs advertised, twenty-six of them claimed to be more effective than they were, and in five of the advertisements the side-effects of the drug being advertised were completely overlooked. Professor Wade expressed his views with these words, '. . . As I look at the current advertisements for these drugs I cannot but feel shame; partly I am disturbed that the pharmaceutical industry should use advertisements more suitable for cosmetics than for drugs, but mainly I am ashamed that such advertisements should be successful in influencing members of a learned profession.'

Both the medical profession and the general public have been led to believe that the pharmaceutical companies are devoted to combating disease, but when I asked a leading personality why the industry was allowed to get away with misleading advertisements of the type described by Professor Wade, and why there were not screams of protest from medical researchers, I was given an answer which I found disturbing:

> What the layman does not appreciate is that the doctors who are in the best position to take them, the drug companies, to task are those who are conducting research projects in hospitals and independent laboratories, and they cannot voice their complaints or doubts too loudly because the pharmaceutical industry donates a lot of money to the research programmes they are doing, and without the money from them they would be unable to continue.

And that was only touching the tip of the iceberg as far as the power of the drug companies is concerned. For there is at least one story which shows there have been occasions when a pharmaceutical company has tried to buy a new medical discovery, which might have benefited millions of people, with the intention of suppressing it.

The late Professor Paul Niehans became famous, or infamous depending upon one's viewpoint, for his Cell Therapy, which he claimed could rejuvenate those parts of the body which had been affected by degenerative disorders. Included among his more illustrious patients was Pope Pius XII, who had been given up by his own physicians as they felt they could do nothing more for him, but who regained his health and strength after being treated by Niehans. The Pope expressed his gratitude by publicly blessing the treatment. Other patients who are said to have benefited are Charlie Chaplin the actor, former President Dwight Eisenhower, Sir Winston Churchill, President de Gaulle, former German Chancellor Konrad Adenaeur, the writer Somerset Maugham, the Duke and Duchess of Windsor, etc.

Niehans found a method of treating diabetes with cells taken from an animal pancreas, and in 1967 he told Peter Stephan, the director of the Cell Therapy Clinic in London, that a pharmaceutical company had approached him to purchase the patent of his diabetic cell preparations A and B. Initially Niehans agreed to the sale, with the proviso that the company purchasing the production rights would actually produce them instead of buying the manfacturing rights to prevent a competitor from putting the preparations on to the market.

As the unnamed manufacturer was interested in buying the production rights it might have been deduced that the company felt it had a definite therapeutic value in the treatment of diabetes. However, as it made and marketed large quantities of insulin, and the Niehans preparations would have replaced this, the company refused to accept the Professor's condition. But they did return to Lausanne at a later date with a counterproposal to the effect that they would still be interested in going into production if it could be agreed that it was produced in a diluted form, thereby ensuring that diabetic patients would still need insulin.

Niehans rejected the offer, and found he had made a powerful enemy. When he entered into an agreement with a small drug company to make up his diabetic cell preparations a larger manufacturer bought up its smaller competitor, and then refused to continue assisting Niehans.

According to Peter Stephan the smear campaign against Niehans continued unabated. Publishers were told that if they were to print any complimentary details of his Cell Therapy the pharmaceutical industry would cease to co-operate with them in future, and that would have meant an immense loss of revenue through the withdrawal of large paid advertisements which medical journals depend upon for survival. Also, and I continue quoting the same source, hospitals were given research grants on the sole condition that the hospitals did not teach or allow any members of the staff to use Niehans' therapy.[5]

All this does not mean that the drug companies are in themselves unethical and unnecessary. They are caught up in their own momentum, and the doctors are being caught up too, so that in the end the overspill of drug abuse has been harmful to all concerned. For as Professor Wade (now at Birmingham University) said, 'There is increasing evidence that the introduction of psychotropic drugs [those chemical preparations which are used to help people overcome nervous and stress conditions, now amounting to nearly fifty million prescriptions a year] may adversely affect the quality of medical practice. It is easier to

C

scribble on a prescription pad than spend a long and difficult session with a patient uncovering the reasons for the psychosomatic conditions . . .'

What Professor Wade is saying is that the General Practitioner can be overworked and take drug-prescribing as an easier way out. That this is already happening cannot be doubted. Chronic sufferers from nervous conditions are often given a prescription for a large number of pills to save the doctor's time in having to see them at regular intervals. This policy has been criticized by the President of the Pharmaceutical Society of Great Britain, Mr John Kerr, in these words, 'With great respect to our medical colleagues, we as pharmacists see no justification for the considerable quantities of highly potent drugs, and drugs of abuse, that are sometimes prescribed today.' In those instances where over-prescribing does not happen, there is a strong tendency for the patient who needs a regular prescription to telephone the surgery and ask the receptionist to get a repeat prescription which can be collected without seeing the doctor.

Dr Frank Wells, a GP in Ipswich, is one of the leaders who is breaking away from the national trend. At his instigation his colleagues in Ipswich in 1958 decided to cut down the amount of amphetamines being handed out, and by November 1959 the operation had been so successful that there was not a single amphetamine held in stock by local chemists. They then turned their attention to barbiturates, and found that 40 per cent of the patients taking this drug no longer needed to take it for the originally prescribed illness – mostly insomnia. The patients had simply got into the habit of taking it. Today the number of barbiturate prescriptions has been reduced to 50 per cent of the former level, and six out of every ten patients who were helped to change over to a safer drug no longer require any sleeping pills at all. Looking at the field of tranquillizers, which are being swallowed daily in massive amounts, and by some people for year after year, Dr Wells says, 'I defy anyone to say that stress lasts that long,' and in keeping with his statement he will only give a 10 to 14 day supply of tranquillizers. When they have been consumed he sees the patient again to reassess the situation, and if a repeat prescription is necessary at the end of each month a further appraisal is made. In this way Dr Wells is able to claim that the rapid upward spiralling of prescribing tranquillizers, which is evident in Britain and the United States, is 'not happening in Ipswich'.

So far it may appear that I have laid all the blame for internal drug pollution upon the shoulders of the medical profession, and this would be unfair as patients too must take some of the responsibility. When they read of a new 'wonder' drug which has just come on to the medical market, usually as a result of the manufacturing pharmaceutical company informing the science or medical editors of newspapers and magazines of its latest product, people flock to their practictioner virtually demanding they be given the new drug. Of course, patients have been well and truly conditioned into expecting newer and better miracle pills to solve all their ills like a magic wand. To counter this the head of the US Food and Drug Administration said early in 1973 that doctors must now start refusing to give their patients drugs upon demand if the American drug-abuse problem is to be overcome.

What he suggested is excellent advice, but what he did not say is that a vital prerequisite must be a stricter control over the non-prescription drugs which are readily available in chemists and drug stores everywhere. These synthetic compounds, meant to cure all minor ailments, are just as much a part of the internal pollution problem as the drugs available only on prescription.

Nor did the head of the Food and Drug Administration dwell upon the extensive use of synthetic chemicals used to give added colour, taste and vitamins to the food being eaten daily, although such practice compounds the hazard to health of every man and woman.

To try and list the foodstuffs that are affected by chemical additives would require a book in itself. The food coming from farms and orchards springs from soil which has been treated by chemical fertilizers, and then sprayed with chemicals to kill pests. The flour in bread is treated with chemicals to give it a better colour, carrots are given artificial colouring to make them look more attractive to the purchaser, and most if not all canned foods contain various chemical preservatives. In the latter category, magnesium salts used in canning peas and curing meats have merited the attention of the Department of Social Medicine of Birmingham University, and the study which the Department carried out showed there are positive associations between the magnesium salts and the subsequent occurrence of anencephalus, congenital brain abnormality.

Continuing this line of thought further, in 1972, Dr A. McLean of University College Hospital Medical School, speaking at a conference organized by the British Association for Social Responsibility in Science, said, 'The food industry may now be in the position of the tobacco industry 50 years ago – selling the customer a product of unknown hazard.' He continued by saying that the food industry had made reasonable tests to ensure that the additives it was using did not cause those eating the products to drop dead, but despite all the controls and efforts the industry had no idea of the long-term effects of the chemicals it was using. He also said both cancer and coronary disease were strongly linked to diet, and 'At the moment we have no guarantee at all of the safety of our foods, and it is only if we begin to do long-term epidemiological studies that we can tackle the long-term diseases.'

While it is agreed that the food industry takes all conceivable steps to ascertain that none of the chemicals it employs are sufficiently toxic to cause death, there is no way for the industry to know exactly what foods the customer will eat or how much of any one food; and therefore it is impossible to foretell which chemicals, and how much of them, will collect in the bloodstream and have to be processed by the liver. This could be very important, because there are a number of medical men who believe that many of our present-day illnesses stem from internal pollution, and that when the bloodstream becomes poisoned by alien chemical substances the finely tuned body-defence mechanisms break down under the strain. If they are correct, it could mean that the drugs we take, when combined with the amount of synthetic chemicals ingested in food, are more dangerous than the illnesses the drugs are meant to treat.

3

Alternative Medicine

Exactly how many people are now rejecting allopathic medicine – the term 'allopathic' being a name given to currently accepted or so-called orthodox medicine by Dr Samuel Hahnemann, 1755–1843 – and going to consult alternative medical practitioners is unknown, although a suggested figure for Britain is more than one million a year. While this and any other figure must be highly speculative, owing to the diversity of therapies and therapists comprising the alternative medical field, there is ample evidence to show that the practitioners who adhere to systems other than the generally accepted, and who can therefore be referred to as being 'heterodox', are thriving; their consulting-rooms are constantly full.

A few typical examples will show the current swing to alternative medicine.

In the city of Liverpool an acupuncturist has a waiting-list of patients which will keep him fully occupied for the next fourteen months, and that is without any further new enquiries being made.

A consultant medical herbalist in Lancashire had to refuse appointments to more than 2,000 people last year, and a thriving medical herbalist's practice in the Midlands has more than 30,000 people on its books.

A friend of mine recently developed a bad back, and when he tried to make an appointment to see the local osteopath he was told by the receptionist that the osteopath could not make any further appointments for the next three and a half months as he was fully booked.

One homeopath in the south of England told me he was working flat out, and was looking for a junior partner to assist him.

And this new cloak of respectability which the public has bestowed upon the former fringe therapist was partially acknowledged by Dr Richard Mackarness, a psychiatrist, in an article he wrote for the medical weekly *General Practitioner* under the heading, 'The Empirical Basis for Fringe Medicine'.[1]

If orthodox medicine was good for all ailments, fringe medicine would not flourish as it does. . . . Fringe medicine may be defined as therapeutic practices not in accord with the current, locally accepted system of medicine.

The areas covered by most fringe practitioners are those which mainly concern the GP: physiologically reversible conditions like asthma, migraine and the functional disorders, both mental and physical, rather than things with established pathology, such as cancer, coronary thrombosis, and massive infections which take the patient into hospital.

Although Dr Mackarness implies the heterodox practitioner has little to offer in the case of pathological disorders such as cancer, etc., this would be strongly disputed, as later chapters in this book will attempt to show.

However, leaving that point to one side until later, one must note that the doctor in his article countered a major criticism often levelled against alternative medicine by his orthodox colleagues that the heterodox healer cannot explain in a scientific manner how the treatment works, and therefore it should be disregarded as being mumbo-jumbo. Dr Mackarness explained that there is 'a much wider and more acceptable way of looking at fringe medicine: effective treatment with an empirical basis', and he pointed out that many of the treatments currently being used by orthodox practitioners were empirically based, such as ECT – Electro-Convulsive Therapy – and digoxin and trinitrin in cases of cardiac disorders, but they continued to be used because there was empirical evidence to show that they were effective.

All this indicates that there is a positive swing away from

allopathic medicine, but it fails to show what lies behind it; what the underlying motivation is.

In the course of talking to people about this phenomenon on both sides of the Atlantic Ocean, I realized there has always been a group of people who have thought that nature holds the cure for all illnesses, and have therefore used the 'natural' or drugless therapist rather than a drug-prescribing allopathic doctor. But this former minority has had its ranks swollen by those reacting to the threat of pollution to future life on this planet, who now feel there has to be a return to a more natural life-style; a return to nature's ways.

Young people who adhere to an alternative society, the former hippies, flower people, etc., have also carried their revolt against materialism into the medical sphere; and they now reject orthodox medicine as being a part of a cancerous society which denies the needs of the individual in favour of those of an élite.

But the most striking facet of this revolt is found in the allopathic doctor's surgery, and the way patients have been treated.

There has been a long tradition of secrecy in orthodox medicine, and this has led to patients being treated as if they were morons by doctors refusing to discuss their cases with them, and not telling them what was wrong or what the treatment being prescribed consisted of and what it was meant to accomplish. And while that paternalistic, autocratic manner may have been ideal for the Middle Ages, when the doctor had to protect the ingredients of his secret potions in order to bolster his prestige, today it is seen as an affront to the patients' intelligence.

Writing in the now defunct herbal medicine journal, *Health from Herbs,* one of Britain's best known practitioners of herbal – botanic – medicine, Captain Frank Roberts, MC, MNIMH, summed up the effects of non-communication in the surgery. 'Time without number patients have come to me and said: "I am consulting you because my doctor will never tell me what is wrong with me. I'm getting so worried. I am certain that I have something so serious that he won't tell me what it is." I have had patients come to me with simple piles or an anal fissure, and, because they have never been *told* what was wrong, they had worried themselves really ill thinking they had cancer of the rectum and that the information was being withheld from them . . .'[2]

Where this type of professional secrecy becomes more marked is when a patient is referred to a GP to see a specialist, and at the end of the examination is told, 'I will sent a report to your doctor, and he will inform you as to my findings.' Naturally it could be stated that this is medical etiquette, and it may well be; but patients have no concern for any ethics involved, they want to know as quickly as possible what is wrong, and feel entitled to be given the information as, after all, they are the people most involved.

Finally there is the feeling, 'My doctor isn't interested in getting down to the root of my problem and finding out what is wrong with me; all he does is give me pills, and they solve nothing.' And this patient-reaction is interesting because it is a reversal of a criticism many orthodox doctors use to discredit alternative medical practitioners.

Time and time again members of the registered medical profession have openly stated that it is dangerous to go and see heterodox therapists as they are both untrained and unqualified, and owing to their lack of knowledge tend to treat symptoms rather than getting down to the real cause. This symptom-treatment, they maintain, borders upon being a criminal act of negligence, for if symptom-removal is practised the undetected cause could result in the patient being even more seriously ill.

Now the boot appears to be on the other foot. For while researching this book I repeatedly asked the herbalists, naturopaths, osteopaths, chiropractors and homeopaths what specific remedies they would prescribe for various specific conditions such as asthma. All of them, without exception, told me they did not practise that type of medicine. They would all conduct a rigid examination of the patient; take a complete medical history; find out about the patient's home, work and social background, and only when all this information had been collected, and not before, would they attempt to make up a prescription or a course of treatment. In other words, unlike their orthodox colleagues, they continue to practise medicine in the orthodox manner summed up in the Italian medical proverb, 'If you do not know the origin of the illness, your medicine is rarely any good.'

I asked a prominent British osteopath and naturopath, Mr Sidney Rose-Neil, what his reaction was to being considered a lay or unqualified practitioner, and he was quick to take umbrage.

'I am not a lay-practitioner. Neither am I unqualified,' Mr Rose-Neil countered. 'I am qualified in my particular discipline. And when doctors use those derogatory terms, what they are really saying is that I am a non-registered practitioner; that I am not listed on the medical register; but I will challenge any of them to prove I am unqualified.'

Another unregistered practitioner, this time a manipulative therapist, also got annoyed when I asked him the same question. He told me, 'I have made a prolonged, in-depth study of my subject, and because I have been forced into a defensive position, owing to the outdated attitude of many members of the medical profession which regards me as unqualified, I have to know more than anyone who is qualified. For if something goes wrong when I am treating a patient I have not got the Medical Defence Union and the magical letters MD after my name to protect me; therefore I am much more knowledgeable than my orthodox medical counterpart.'

That there is antagonism between orthodox and heterodox medicine cannot be denied, yet it must not be overlooked that much of the orthodox opposition is emotive rather than scientific. There is a tendency among registered practitioners to dismiss any form of alternative therapy administered by a non-registered therapist as being downright quackery, while it is acceptable if the alternative therapy is carried out by one of their own ranks. It may sound ridiculous and bordering upon Alice in Wonderland, but it is true! I have met it in the course of my own work.

Over the years I have held courses throughout the British Isles to train doctors and dentists how to use hypnosis in their respective practices. What I taught during the seminars was acceptable to a leading registered medical exponent of hypnosis, who told many of his colleagues he would have me on his lecuring staff if only I were 'qualified' – on either the medical or dental register. Yet the fact that I, an unregistered practitioner, should be running courses for registered men and women has been condemned in certain quarters, and suggestions have been made to the effect that only registered practitioners should be allowed to do this. The knowledge I had to offer was disregarded, and this situation became patently ludicrous after I had held a weekend advanced course in Leeds a few years ago, dealing with the aetiology of neurosis, and methods which could be used to unearth the causes underlying the presenting symptomatology.

One of the people attending the advanced course subsequently went on a medically approved course in psychiatry, and when he began to expound the various psychodynamic concepts I had outlined in Leeds earlier, the senior lecturer conducting the psychiatric course was impressed and asked if he would give a full lecture to the other students. Naturally he was pleased to do so, and the students thought his contribution was valuable.

As we are good friends, when I was told about his giving my lecture virtually verbatim and the approval it met with, I was amused. His knowledge and experience was limited, but acceptable, whereas my own was not. Yet doctors and dentists still telephone me and ask for my advice on how to treat their patients!

Again it could be said that I have an axe to grind and that therefore I cannot be sufficiently objective about the controversy raging between accepted and alternative medicine, and that I may allow my emotions to sway me in favour of heterodox medical practice. This is incorrect. My only concern is that people who are ill should get help, the best help possible, irrespective of whether the therapist is registered or unregistered. For far too long irrational behaviour has prevented this, as evidenced some years ago in the United States when a prominent member of the American Medical Association, Dr Morris Fishbein, was asked by an irate judge why he, Dr Fishbein, condemned the Hoxsey herbal treatment for cancer, a treatment which lawyers acting for the orthodox medical profession had previously conceded in a court of law did cure certain cancers. Dr Fishbein lamely explained: *it is customary for doctors to oppose unorthodox methods . . .*

4

The Oldest Medicine - Herbalism

'We are specialists in curing the incurables.' This is how consulting medical herbalist, Mr John Hyde of Leicester, assessed the work of medical herbalists in Britain.

It sounded dramatic, but the reason he gave for his statement was that the patients he and his colleagues had to see had already been through the entire orthodox medical process; they had seen their doctors, and various specialists, had tests and treatment galore, and in certain cases been hospitalized; nevertheless at the end of it all they had been classified as incurable. 'If this had not happened, and their doctor or the specialist had been able to help them, they would never have arrived to see us,' Mr Hyde expounded. 'Our whole life is spent looking at the long-term diseases that the doctor and the general orthodox profession have found they are unable to cope with.'

I asked him if he could give me a typical example to back up his claim, and he quoted the case of a lady in her fifties whose job necessitated that she be on her feet throughout the day, working in the open air and in all weather from five am until six pm. She arrived at the Hyde Clinic with varicose ulcers, both legs badly ulcerated, with ulcers verging upon the post thrombotic almost through to the bone, an inch deep in the bed, while two of the ulcers on the left leg had a very rodent look about them.

Prior to going to see Mr Hyde she had undergone operations and skin grafts, but they were all of no avail. When she arrived at the clinic and removed the bandages the room literally stank to high heaven with the reek of putrid flesh, and the ulceration went from the foot to above the knees on both legs with hardly a square inch of normal skin being seen. Mr Hyde's description was, 'She looked like a leprosy candidate,' and in his opinion this was the worst case of varicose ulcers he had ever seen.

The treatment was chosen carefully, and it was two years before healing began to be evident, but at the end of the third year both legs were completely healed, and at present the lady has nothing more than a slight, whitish scar down her left leg, while on the right leg there is no indication of where the ulceration has been.

According to Mr Hyde, who in addition to being a consultant herbalist is the Public Relations Officer for the National Institute of Medical Herbalists, and other herbalists I talked to, for every illness known to man nature has provided an answer in the shape of one herb or a combination of herbs.

But how did mankind find the herbs which had curative powers? The answer I received was that the birth of herbalism came to our primitive ancestors at the dawn of civilization through their observation of the behaviour of animals who were sick, and of the fact that they would, depending upon the illness, go and eat certain plants or grasses, and that these would in the majority of cases cure them. Primitive man decided to eat the same plants and grasses when he was ill, and that, according to legend, is how herbalism came into being.

The story had a pleasant ring to it, yet it could hardly be accepted as a fact as there was no proof to substantiate it. Or at least there wasn't, as far as I was concerned, until I read about one of America's most famous, or notorious, herbalists, Dr Harry M. Hoxsey, ND, a naturopathic physician of Dallas, Texas. Dr Hoxsey said that his great-grandfather, John Hoxsey, had discovered a herbal remedy for treating cancer in about 1840, after watching the behaviour of a prize stallion he owned in Illinois.

The horse had developed a sore on the ankle that soon spread to the entire hoof. A veterinary surgeon diagnosed it as cancer, and recommended that the horse be destroyed, as it would die anyway because there was nothing which could be done to cure it. John Hoxsey was loath to kill his prize animal, and decided to wait a while before he did anything.

To his delight the horse did not die. After it had been left to pasture and to its own devices for some weeks, Hoxsey found that the ugly sore was beginning to heal rather than to get worse. Unable to accept what he thought he saw, he decided to watch the animal closely to see if the horse's natural instinct was leading it to find its own cure.

He noticed that the horse used to go to a particular part of the field, and that it would meticulously and regularly eat certain herbs that were growing there, and as the weeks passed Hoxsey became positive that the cancer was remitting. He was correct, and within a few months the cancer had dried out and fallen away, leaving clean, healthy scar-tissue where the malignant growth had formerly been.

Impressed and intrigued by the stallion's selection of herbs, John Hoxsey collected them, and began to experiment by brewing them into various concoctions, which he tried out on other cancerous animals. At first it was all trial and error, but eventually he developed two herbal formulae – one for internal and the other for external use – and these proved, at least as far as Hoxsey and those who benefited were concerned, effective in the treatment of cancer in animals and then in human beings.[1]

Nor does the reader have to rely upon historical data to show how his ancestors may well have discovered the remedial effects of herbs in combating illness. If you have ever owned a dog and taken it for a walk when it was ill, you will have noticed that it spontaneously ate certain grasses which it would ignore when it was well. The dog seems to know instinctively what will make it better!

A fact supporting the story that this herbal system of medicine arose through observation of sick animals, rather than through a lucky chance-find by an individual living in a specific country or area is the fact that plants containing healing powers have not been confined to any one geographical location. On the contrary, wherever people lived herbal medicine was a part of their lives.

Prior to 2,000 BC herbal medicine in China had become a definite system of medicine. In Egypt it is known from papyrus documents which are still in existence that in the year 2,000 BC there were more than a thousand herbal physicians who, having given up trying to cure illnesses by magical incantations, made an exhaustive study of the healing effects embodied in herbs, and compiled various formulae for treating a number of diseases of the stomach, as well as deafness and nervous conditions. And in the British Museum in London there are records of herbal remedies from the time of the Sumerian civilization which were originally in the library of the King of Assyria (668–626 BC).

As it would require a complete volume to give a world history of herbalism I have decided to limit this short survey to Europe, as European herbal medicine as a science can be traced back to Hippocrates, the father of medicine both orthodox and heterodox.

Again there are records to show that Hippocrates was summoned to see the King of Macedon, who had fallen ill. He saw his royal patient and diagnosed the illness as melancholia, the equivalent to modern depression, and treated it successfully with a herbal compound.

In the course of his life Hippocrates listed 400 herbal remedies which he used in his practice of medicine, and a member of the National Institute of Medical Herbalists informed me that a third of them are still being currently used by consultant herbalists.

Here in Britain herbalism has long been a part of everyday life, and some of the plants which grow wild in the fields and hedgerows have names which refer to the way they have been used in herbal medicine, and to the effects they have on certain parts of the body. An illustration can be found in the plant *agrimony,* more commonly known as *liverwort,* the word 'wort' being Anglo-Saxon for 'plant'. It was given the name because it was thought to help cure liver conditions, and research recently undertaken by the British Herbal Medicine Association has confirmed it has a diuretic effect, and its use is indicated for 'Diarrhoea in children, mucous colitis. . . . Urinary incontinence. Cystitis.'[2] J. Hewlett-Parsons, Founder and Director of Studies of the General Council and Register of Consultant Herbalists, recommended in his book *Herbs, Health and Healing,*[3] that liverwort be used as one of the ingredients in a herbal compound for treating the liver complaint jaundice.

All too often these thousands of years of herbal history are dismissed as unimportant, and the names of famous herbalists such as Mr Jesse Boot of Nottingham, later the first Lord Trent and the founder of one of Britain's largest manufacturing, retailing and dispensing multiple chemists, are studiously forgotten. The therapeutic value of herbal remedies is labelled as folk-lore with little more than a placebo effect.

The medical herbalists have learned to live with the innuendoes and derision aimed at them, and a herbal practitioner gave me some of the reasons for this denigration:

'Until recently it has been part of modern mythology to believe that everything which is modern must be better than anything which has gone before, and this has applied to medicine. Yet now the situation is changing. People are beginning to accept there is nothing wrong with medicines which have a proven value, as ours has. And let me put the record straight: our remedies worked in the past and they work now. People are beginning to realize that herbal remedies, with their proven background over the centuries, have continued to be used (a) because they are safe to use, and (b) because of their efficacy. Compare our record with that of drugs which have only been on the market for a few months and hailed as *wonder drugs,* when there is a killer backlash, and they have to be withdrawn. This has never happened to a herbal remedy, and no herbal remedy has had to be withdrawn, because they have proved to be safe and effective.'

He also reminded me that the allopathic doctor also owes a lot to herbalism.

I asked him to explain what he meant, and he told me the history of the aspirin.

In the days of ancient Greece Hippocrates would treat fevers or minor aches and pains with extracts or infusions of willow-bark (*salix nigra*), and for hundreds of years after him people in Britain would make and drink a 'willow tea' whenever they were struck with aches or fevers; in the same way North American Indians used a similar willow tea for rheumatism long before the first settlers set foot upon the North American continent.

The Latin name for the willow tree is *salix,* and it was from this that the name salicylic acid, or aspirin, was derived when the compound was chemically synthesized by chemists in 1840. From the time the aspirin was chemically created the orthodox medical profession saw it as the best and safest means of giving relief to those of their patients with rheumatism – that is until 1949, when synthetic adrenal hormones, cortisone and ACTH appeared on the medical market as the ultimate weapons in the war against rheumatism and arthritis. For a period the new chemical preparations lived up to the claims made on their behalf. People who had been incapacitated for years found they had a greater physical mobility and freedom from pain. But then came the backlash in the form of side-effects which made doctors reluctant to use it unless it was imperative. So they had to resort to aspirin again.

Digitalis, widely used for heart conditions, is derived from the foxglove plant; the drug serpasil, which is beneficial in treating high blood-pressure and certain nervous disorders, comes from the plant *rauwolfia serpentina;* strophantine the heart drug, emetine used in amoebic dysentry, and picrotoxine, a stimulator in cases of barbiturate poisoning, are only a few more of the drugs used in allopathic medicine which really belong to the herbal pharmacopeia.

When the question of rheumatism and arthritis cropped up in the conversation I made a note to ask Mr John Hyde what success he and his colleagues had had in this field, as it was still considered by the orthodoxy as a chronic, incurable ailment.

Mr Hyde assured me that he personally, and all consultant herbalists, had achieved good results in this curative area. 'Our treatment aims at the complete elimination of the disease rather than being palliative, which is all the orthodox practitioner can do,' he emphasized. 'In fact our treatment has to be curative, because we do not have any palliative remedies.'

As there are millions of people throughout the world crippled with rheumatism and arthritis I requested he tell me more about the actual herbal treatment involved.

The herbalist starts out from an entirely different viewpoint from the orthodox physician, in as much as he believes that both rheumatoid- and osteo-arthritis are caused by faults within the metabolic process, and that they stem from faulty nutrition, faults in the bloodstream, and faults in renal clearance, from liver disorders and associated conditions. Another point of divergence is that the herbalist doesn't attempt to eliminate or ease the pain which goes with the disease.

The first thing the herbalist does when commencing treatment with a rheumatic patient is to get him or her to forget about taking pain-killers, and to start observing nature's laws. 'If nature doesn't want you to walk on that bad knee,' the patient is told, 'then don't walk on it. Rest. If you get pain, limit movement or stop, as the body does not want you to use it.' Of course this is not always practicable. Some people still have to go to work, housewives still have to cook and clean the house, and mothers have to look after their children. In these instances the patient is permitted to use a small amount of pain-killing preparations when it is imperative, but is urged to follow nature's advice whenever possible.

To the herbal practitioner the pain is an alarm bell, a warning signal, and should not be considered as unimportant. Therefore if a patient gets pain from an arthritic joint it is considered by the herbalists to be irresponsible to administer cortisone or an analgesic such as aspirin, because the latter is acidic and in the long term will build up in the bloodstream and make the affected joint ten times worse.

Once the patient embarks upon herbal treatment the practitioner's aim is to increase the blood supply to the diseased joint, and to increase not only the volumetric supply, but also the quality of the blood; then to increase the deposition of new tissue for repairing the affected area, and to step up the discharge of internal debris to be taken away from the diseased area. Bowel and kidney action is increased to clear the system of toxins that have built up in it, and dietary advice is given to ensure the patient keeps clear of acids, and the more acid-producing meats like pork.

Listening to this therapeutic procedure, I thought that it sounded very much the same sort of treatment, minus the herbal remedies, that a naturopath would undertake; and I asked Mr

D

Hyde if this was where the herbalist and the naturopath met on common ground. He wasn't happy about the comparison. In his opinion the dietary regimes the naturopath would prescribe are inadequate. 'They will do good in some cases, and in milder cases of arthritis they may clear it, but the dietary approach is insufficient because there are so many other factors in the body that have to be taken into account.' However, he qualified that by adding, 'It could be said that by administering a herbal medicine one is only following a dietary regime, because taking it down to basic principles a herb is food, and the herbalist could be said to be simply giving a food supplement.'

But leaving aside the differences separating the naturopath and the herbalist and concentrating upon the treatment of rheumatism, it was easy for me to accept the theory underlying the therapy. Yet did it work?

For a middle-aged male whose case history I was able to examine, it certainly did.

He had suffered from rheumatoid arthritis so badly that he was unable to continue his work in the building trade. He was virtually a cripple, having to be dressed when he got up in the morning – and even that was a painful experience – and to be carried from one place to another, being unable to drive his car. Orthodox treatments had been tried without success.

After he had been carried into the herbalist's consulting rooms, a long, painstaking case history was undertaken, including what can only be called a personality profile. This is always considered as most important, for if the patient had other organic disabilities certain herbs would be contra-indicated. For instance, ragwort is recommended by the *British Herbal Pharmacopeia* for use in rheumatoid arthritis, but has to be avoided if the patient has a liver disorder.

This particular male patient was given his medication and suggested diet, and within four months he was able to walk without using a stick. Two months after that he was driving his car again, and a little more than a year later he was back at work, experiencing hardly any discomfort.

Going further into the work of the herbalist, let us consider two of the most common complaints afflicting people in modern society: insomnia, which can lead to addiction to sleeping pills and the occasional accidental overdose; and stress disorders, anxiety and depression, plus certain phobias, that in the majority of cases also require repeated prescriptions of tranquillizers and anti-depressants.

In my own practice the records show the insomniac and the stress sufferer to comprise more than 90 per cent of my clients. I was therefore interested to find out if herbalists had to cope with a similarly high proportion, and, if they did, I wondered how they tackled the problems.

Insomnia is a problem which they are always meeting, and like psychotherapists they do not treat the actual presenting symptom. They are more interested in trying to locate the possible causes for it. When did it start, and what was the physical and mental state of the patient at the outset? Is it mentally based? Is it the inability to relax? Is it somatically based – in the body? Is it some sort of rigour or fine tremor of the limbs, an involuntary jerk, that awakens the patient? Is it based in the nervous system? Or is it a mixture of several of these? Is it due to indigestion, a desire to urinate, an unsatisfactory love or sexual life, or does it come from emotional stress? These are the questions the herbalist wants answers to before attempting to alleviate the symptom.

There are many remedies the herbalist uses to restore normal sleep patterns, and he finds he has no difficulties unless the patient is already taking barbiturates or other sleeping pills. If this is so, the herbalist has to find herbs to adequately replace the drug, then institute a gradual change-over, perhaps by reducing one pill at a time, as this allows the herbalist to ensure the best herb or herbs have been selected for the patient.

Those suffering from stress are weaned away from the drug and onto the herbal replacement – and there are various groups which can be prescribed – and the patient has to be prepared to continue the herbal treatment for some length of time to make certain all the toxic effects of the drug have been eliminated from the body, and to be sure the herbal treatment has taken effect.

Consultant herbalists have found in their experience that if the condition is of long standing the patient should continue taking the herbal preparations for something in the region of six months, and then the dosage is gradually reduced until the person has had two weeks without taking any medication. When that stage of the treatment is reached the patient is given a complete check-up (blood, urine, heart, blood pressure, etc.) and the results are compared with the results of the same tests carried out at the initial visit. By comparing the results of the two series of tests the herbalist assesses if the patient has been treated effectively, and if further treatment is necessary.

As I felt it was my self-appointed role to play the Devil's Advocate, there were three aspects of both treatments which left me with questions I felt had to be answered.

How safe are the herbal remedies being used?

From what various herbalists have told me, the treatment of the stress-sufferer is long-term; therefore how do their patients react to this, since chemical tranquillizers act more quickly?

Finally, looking at the economics of the treatment, for how long does the practitioner see a patient at the initial consultation? How long would the average treatment take, and what could the cost be?

In answer to my question about possible dangers I was informed that I was speaking of a relative thing, and that one must compare the toxicity of drugs, as formed from synthesized products and chemicals and prescribed by a registered practitioner, with the toxicity of herbal remedies. 'Now, if you are using the word "dangerous" as applied to chemical drugs, in comparison the remedies prescribed by the herbal practitioner are absolutely innocuous as they have no toxicity whatsoever,' I was told by a herbalist. Another consultant herbalist answered the same question slightly differently. 'With chemical drugs you can get iatrogenic illnesses, because the chemical compounds are unnatural. Herbal compounds are natural, and cannot cause iatrogenic diseases.' I took his point. Yet a third herbalist said, 'If you mean, "Can our remedies be harmful?" then we must answer no, providing they are taken as we prescribe. But, if you take too much of anything, castor oil for instance, this can be harmful.'

John Hyde replied to my enquiry about people wanting quick results from their medication. 'Admittedly in this age that we live in everyone wants everything yesterday, and if we have a headache and there is a tablet which will take it away in three minutes obviously we will buy it in preference to the one which will take five minutes. But people are realizing that this is to their detriment – and there is some evidence that doctors are realizing it too – and many patients have said on their second visit, "Mr Hyde, I am already feeling the benefit of the treatment, and I don't mind how long it takes, because now I know you are really getting down to the bottom of it. And once you have put me right I know I won't have to carry on taking pills." The herbalist aims at getting the condition completely cleared, rather than just putting it off.'

From a treatment and cost point of view this must obviously vary from practice to practice. Some herbalists are in solo practice, doing their own dispensing and making up their own tinctures. In such cases the patient will get more than an hour at the initial consultation. Whereas in a group herbal practice dealing with hundreds of patients a week and having its own dispensers, the average time appears to be approximately forty minutes for the new patient, although this depends upon the type of case presenting itself. The next appointment is usually two weeks later and lasts some twenty minutes to half an hour, and the patient is seen each fortnight for the same amount of time until the healing process is noticeable. After that the length between visits is stretched to three weeks, then a month, and finally six weeks. In accumulated time this would take about six months, although that is a generalization as herbalists feel that for every year a patient has had a condition two months are required to eradicate it. As for the cost of the treatment and medicines, these vary. The National Institute of Medical Herbalists has no national policy because overheads vary from practice to practice, but a spokesman thought it would average out at about £1 per week.

What surprises anyone investigating herbalism as a medical system is the diversity of cases the consultant herbalist handles, from the small child to the aged with chronic conditions, but in

Britain the overall image of the herbalist remains far below that of the registered medical practitioner, and for that matter the osteopath.

The oldest association of medical herbalists, the National Institute of Medical Herbalists, has been trying to change this public image and to dissociate itself from the idea that the consultant herbalist runs a herbal shop where people drop in and casually consult the owner about what remedy they need and should buy.

A statement made by an official of the NIMH said:

The National Institute is composed of consultants and practitioners who consult with a patient, and having examined him carefully in every detail by the latest diagnostic techniques, arrive at a diagnosis and base their treatment accordingly. Our members—and there are approximately 200 of them in the British Isles – only prescribe for individual needs.

Now, the shopkeeper who has a mixture for this, that and the other is not a consultant and he does not claim to be. Of course, if a person going into a shop gets relief from the brand or product or whatever the shopkeeper offers them, obviously we would want them to gain relief, but only as long as no one confuses the consulting herbalist with the retailer of herbs. They are two entirely different things. It is rather like suggesting you could equate a doctor of medicine with a lady down at the corner who has a sweetshop; if you ask her to sell you something for a headache – a box of aspirins – she will sell you one, but it does not make her a doctor.

When I have asked doctors to give me their opinion about herbalism and herbalists many of them have criticized the lack of training. There is some truth to this as anyone in Britain can obtain textbooks on herbalism and set himself up as a medical herbalist, but the two main training organizations in the United Kingdom do insist that all would-be herbalists undergo an intensive course.

The National Institute of Medical Herbalists course is of four years duration.

Its curriculum is inclusive of the following courses:

First year
Anatomy, Physiology
Elementary Biology
Elementary Chemistry
Elementary Physics
Theory and Practice of
 Medical Herbalism

Second year
Advanced Anatomy and
 Physiology
Herbal Materia Medica
Symptomatology and Prin-
 ciples of Diagnosis
Pathology

Third year
Nutrition and Dietetics
Differential Diagnosis
Physiomedical Philosophy and
 Materia Medica
Diseases of Women and
 Children
Practical Course:
 Structural Diagnosis and
  Principles, Manipulative
  Treatment

Fourth year
Ethics and Medical Juris-
 prudence
Clinical Psychology and
 Psychosomatic Medicine
Physiomedical Therapeutics
Practical Courses:
 Clinical Pathology and
  Laboratory Diagnosis
 Physical Diagnosis
 Pharmacy
 Clinical training

In the prospectus it sends out to aspiring herbalists the NIMH does state, 'It is not possible to accept students who are living overseas and who are unable to reside in this country for the duration of the course.' This point is stressed because although the four-year course is primarily a correspondence course, it is essential for the new student to attend practical weekend seminars throughout the first two years, and then to be available to work with patients, under the supervision of a qualified practitioner, during the fourth and final year – a clinical training that has to be successfully completed before the student is allowed to sit for the final examination.

Now, as this is being written, the Institute has launched an appeal for money to build a well-equipped college which will train a new generation of consultants in herbal therapy to meet the increasing public demand for local, qualified practitioners. If the appeal is well received, and already many thousands of pounds have been donated, the course would cease to be a correspondence course, and become a full-time four-year training programme. How soon the college will be built is a matter of speculation, but it appears that the Institute is prepared to accept anyone as a student, irrespective of their academic background, provided they can convince members of the Institute's Educational Committee they 'have a sincere interest in the principles and practice of herbal medicine, and . . . have the capacity for study.' Although it does state 'Preference will be given to applicants with GCE 'A' level passes in relevant subjects', it then gives a further academic loophole: that 'suitable applicants with 'O' level passes, including English language, will receive consideration.'

The members of the Institute feel that no one should be barred from becoming a medical herbalist through lack of prior educational opportunities, as family circumstances may have prevented the applicant from continuing with further education when younger. This liberal attitude is welcomed by hundreds of thousands of mature students throughout the world, who are thereby given the opportunity to obtain qualifications they had been barred from earlier. As a leading member of the Institute said, there is a built-in safeguard against any lowering of standards, because if a student has not got the intellectual capabilities to absorb and utilize the knowledge then he will fail to complete the course, either by deciding to drop out on his own initiative, or by being failed by the Institute's examining body. And he assured me the failure rate is high.

The other leading training organization in Britain is the Faculty of Herbal Medicine with its headquarters in Winchester. It was founded twenty-five years ago, to 'provide training in all spheres for students wishing to become qualified Medical Herbalists'. Today it is the official training programme of the General Council and Register of Consultant Herbalists.

Tuition with the Faculty is completed in three ways: by a series of three correspondence courses comprising thirty-seven lessons; by a series of lectures and demonstrations held at the headquarters in Winchester; and finally by practical experience to be gained by working with a member of the Register of Consultant Herbalists.

I asked the founder of the General Council and Register of Consultant Herbalists, J. Hewlett-Parsons, how long the correspondence part of the herbal course would take a student. He told me the length varied according to the time the student could give to studying, and to the student's capabilities. The average was eighteen months, but by those who could give more time it could be completed in six months.

As there is a marked difference between the four-year course offered by the NIMH and the six to eighteen months usually needed to complete the Faculty of Herbal Medicine's programme, I asked Mr Hewlett-Parsons why the anomaly existed. His explanation was that the length of time needed to complete the course was immaterial as the Faculty ensured that, irrespective of the time taken, each student had reached what was considered to be a qualifying standard.

Despite Mr Hewlett-Parsons' answer the time differential is a cause of friction; one group thinks that the shorter course is lowering the standard of the profession, while the other feels that a prolonged course has been unnecessarily concocted in order to imitate the orthodox medical training.

From my own observations both courses could be improved; but under prevailing conditions it has to be admitted that each organization makes every attempt to see their students have sufficient theoretical and practical knowledge to practise herbal medicine, and therefore the charge laid against the consultant herbalists by registered medical practitioners to the effect that they are untrained can be rephrased to mean, 'They are not trained in our methodology of medicine; as a result they cannot be as good as us.'

The same professional antagonism for another system of medicine may well be causing untold suffering, and hampering the progress of the fight against illness. For in the US magazine *Time* dated 15 June 1959, there appeared an item in the medical section entitled 'Herb Hunters' which told of how in the five continents 750 doctors and orthodox medical personnel were collecting plants and folk-lore remedies to see if they could be added to allopathic medical practice. It mentioned the discovery of the drug reserpine from Snake Root, and of the drug ephredrine, which is prepared from a Chinese herb called Ma Hunung, and has been used by Chinese herbal practitioners for 5,000 years. The *Time* article then quoted Dr Alfred Taylor of the University of Texas as saying there was every reason to believe there were many more valuable drugs to be found where these drugs had come from, i.e. from herbs and plants.

On reading *Time* magazine the then Public Relations Officer of the National Institute of Medical Herbalists wrote a letter to the editors of the magazine:

I was interested to read in your magazine on 15 June 1959, under the section Medicine, an account entitled "The Herb Hunters". Mention is made of the herb *Ma Hunung* in the treatment of asthma, and *Rawolfia Serpentaria,* in other words Indian Snake Root, which is useful in Hypertension. These are among many botanical remedies which are used in the treatment of maladies that afflict mankind. In this country the Herbalist is protected by a Royal Charter but in spite of this, medical science lags behind in the progress that could be made if there was some co-operation between the orthodox and un-orthodox medical fraternity. Much human suffering persists in consequence of this lack of liaison ...

... It is ironical when we read of the financial investments made in an endeavour to rediscover the things that are already known. The Herbalist is not given official credit for the work he does; indeed there is not the least doubt that much of the knowledge coveted by the individual Herbalist would be more widely publicised if a greater co-operation was given to this branch of healing arts. Although the Herbalist specialises in the use of botanical medicine he is never consulted when investigation is made into the properties and usage of the natural drugs ...

It is strange that in this modern age great scientists class the Herbalist as a quack. Men will face great danger and expend untold wealth in an endeavour to extort from the witch doctor his secrets, which will ultimately pay dividends to the shareholders of the chemical industry.

There is nothing more humiliating to the *bona fide* Herbalist than to read of a new medical achievement based upon some herb which up to the moment of investigation might have been despised by the very scientists making claim to discovery.[4]

5
Can Herbs Cure Cancer?

As it is illegal in Britain for anyone other than a registered medical practitioner to claim they can successfully treat cancer, it is difficult to obtain a definitive answer to the question, 'Can herbs cure cancer?', especially when the herbalist knows his answer may appear in print. Nevertheless, some herbalists know certain types of cancer have remitted when they have prescribed certain herbal remedies. One gentleman gave me details of a dramatic case history in which a patient had responded well to herbal medicine, but he became reticent when I enquired about the exact ingredients he would use in cases of cancer. He informed me this would depend upon the type of cancer being presented, the location of the malignancy, the extent of the growth, and whether it had spread into other parts of the body. That sounded both a reasonable and a professional approach to this scourge of the twentieth century, yet when I asked if I could quote the case he gave to me, together with his own name, he refused.

Another heterodox practitioner who is using a herbal preparation together with a dietary regime to combat cancer told me of a woman who had been to see him with cancer of the breast, which had spread and reached the point of being inoperable. She was given her herbal remedy and put onto a special diet, and a year later the cancer had remitted. Her own physician was amazed at the progress she had made, and when he too was subsequently diagnosed to have cancer, instead of submitting to the orthodox procedures he presented himself to the heterodox prescriber.

Again, when I asked if I could publish more about his work, as he has a large number of cancer patients, he refused, although he did inform me that part of the treatment comprised the Hoxsey herbal method together with the dietary concept of another American, Dr William Donald Kelley, DDS, MS, of Grapevine, Texas.

I had already written to Dr Kelley after reading his booklet, 'New Hope for Cancer Victims',[1] requesting information about *The Kelley Malignancy Index*, which it is alleged 'determines the presence or absence of cancer, the size and growth rate of the tumor, the location of the tumor mass, prognosis of the treatment, age of the tumor, and the regulation of medication for treatment'. This sounded, if the claims made for it could be substantiated, a tremendous breakthrough since, by future screening of the population, cancer could be detected at inception and be more amenable to treatment.

Instead of receiving an answer to my question I got through the mail a photo-copied circular letter informing me that the Texas Medical Board had an injunction against Dr Kelley's publishing the booklet 'One Answer to Cancer',[2] and owing to recent court actions Dr Kelley was not permitted to talk to anyone on the telephone about his nutritional programmes which he had used to combat cancer, or to talk about his method of detecting cancer.

Fortunately, the licensed physicians working at the former Hoxsey Cancer Clinic in Dallas, Texas, where herbal preparations were used, had a lot to say about their own findings.

In 1953 the editor of the Mexican weekly magazine *Tiempo*, Sr Martin Luis Guzman, went to Texas to investigate the claims of Dr Harry M. Hoxsey, ND, that he could cure cancer by herbal remedies, and Sr Guzman was told by doctors at the clinic:

Our files show that we cure about 85 per cent of external cases and about 25 per cent of internal. In cancer of the breast our cures range from 50 to 60 per cent. We have even cured cases of melanoma (black cancer) which according to most medical texts is 100 per cent fatal. We defy any hospital or cancer specialist to equal that record.

It is all the more remarkable when you consider that the vast majority of patients who come to us are advanced cases, after the disease has already metastasized (spread through the body to other organs), after extensive treatment by surgery, radium, X-ray or a combination of these have failed, many of them after they have already been given up as hopeless by their own doctors.

If we were to get cases in the first stages of the disease, before metastasis and before the knife and radium destroy circulation to the affected parts, we firmly believe we could cure 95 per cent of all external and 50 per cent of all internal cases.

Although those were positive claims and based upon thousands of case histories, Dr Hoxsey did not claim to cure all cases of cancer. He and his colleagues simply stated that the remission rate was higher than that claimed for accepted, orthodox procedures. Yet what is the evidence available to support this?

The only way I found to collect the facts was to trace the history of the Hoxsey herbal treatment, the beginning of which I wrote about in the last chapter. Dr Hoxsey's great-grandfather, John Hoxsey, discovered in the spring of 1840 that one of his prize Percheron horses had developed a sore on the hock, which soon encompassed the entire hoof. The veterinarian called in diagnosed it as cancer, and said it should be shot as there was nothing to cure it.

As described previously, the horse did not die, but, as a result of instinctively selecting a diet of red clover, alfalfa, buckthorn, prickly ash, and a number of other herbs, it recovered.

Having isolated an internal and external treatment John Hoxsey was soon treating cancerous animals from near and far afield, but he always kept his formulae secret, and only on his death-bed did he pass the details on to his son.

It was the original discoverer's grandson, John C. Hoxsey, a breeder of horses on a farm in Illinois, who used this knowledge extensively. Thus when the 1877 Illinois Medical Practices Act became law and permitted anyone who had been practising medicine for six years to become State-licensed, he became Dr John Hoxsey, a veterinary surgeon.

The newly licensed vet moved into the township of Girard to practise, and before long he had people coming to see him, begging him to try the cancer medicines on them. If they worked on animals they reasoned they might work on humans too. For some they did, and Dr John C. Hoxsey found that his people-practice began to outweigh his veterinarian one, and although he did not attempt to publicize what he was doing, news quickly spread by word of mouth.

This placed him in a dangerous position. Not being a licensed physician he could face criminal charges if he continued to treat human patients, but he managed to circumvent the problem by initially working under the supervision of a licensed physician, Dr W. W. Dunton, and then under Dr A. A. Simmons.

In 1915 he had an accident which led to a long and severe illness and drained away all his capital, necessitating that his son Harry go and work in the mines to help support the family.

Four years later, when he was about to die, John C. Hoxsey called his son to him, and made him memorize the herbal formulae, and a few days later he died of erysipelas.

Harry Hoxsey was eighteen years old when he received his legacy and with it the problems which were to remain with him for decades to come.

Young Harry had always wanted to be a doctor of medicine; only the decline in the family finances prevented him going through college and medical school, but the dream remained. Accordingly, when people visited him asking if he would treat them with the family herbal medicines, he refused; that is, until a prominent local businessman, a Mr Larkin arrived at his home.

Mr Larkin's lip and jaw were a giant running sore that doctors had diagnosed as cancer and beyond aid. He asked Harry Hoxsey to help him. At first he refused, but then acceded to the request, hoping his patient would not die as he would then be in severe trouble.

At his next visit Larkin brought with him a director of the

local bank, who had a sore on his right temple which a doctor in Springfield, Illinois, had told him was cancer and incurable. When they returned for their next treatment they brought Hoxsey yet another patient, this time a man whose hand was completely cancerous. And that was the start of his real use of the Hoxsey cancer treatment.

Then he met the forty-five-year-old wife of a local farmer, a Mrs Stroud, who had cancer of the left breast; it was too advanced to be amputated as it had metastasized. Instead the hospital gave her radium and X-ray treatment, but it was to no avail, and she was finally sent home to die. Hoxsey told her husband that it was too late even for him, that there was little chance of him being of any help. Mr Stroud asked him to try, and to the surprise of everyone, Hoxsey included, Mrs Stroud began to recover. In 1956 she was still alive at the good age of 76 years.

A Dr Maximillian Meinhardt, the head of a sanatorium, heard of Hoxsey's work, and asked him if he would treat some of his patients at the sanatorium, under his supervision. He agreed and treated ten people, who responded. And it was there he met a Dr Miller, who, although extremely sceptical in the beginning, nevertheless after meeting the patients Hoxsey had been treating in Taylorville and discussing their individual case histories with their doctors, put a proposition to the heterodox healer. His idea was that he would establish a clinic in Taylorville where he would be the medical director, and Harry Hoxsey his technical assistant. The doctor would examine and diagnose all the patients in order to build up a solid file of case histories to support the efficacy of the treatment, and to protect Hoxsey from being accused of practising medicine without a licence. It was further proposed that the Hoxsey formulae would remain secret until they were recognized by the profession as valuable weapons in the fight against cancer; and that $300 was to be the maximum charge for the complete treatment. Should a patient be unable to pay then he or she would be treated without charge.

Hoxsey talked it over with his friends in Taylorville and they agreed to help finance the new clinic. On 1 March 1924, the clinic opened at 401, Park Street, Taylorville.

Within a few months the number of patients arriving at the clinic had grown to such an extent that the premises had become too small; and they were looking for a larger building when a local businessman, Mr L. Everhard, informed them that if half of what he had heard about their work was correct the future clinic should not be in Taylorville but in a large medical centre. Mr Everhard's suggestion was that he telephone Dr Malcolm Harris of the Alexian Brothers Hospital, and President of the American Medical Association, and ask Dr Harris to give Hoxsey and Dr Miller a chance to prove they have a cure for certain types of cancer. Naturally Hoxsey was pleased with the idea, and both of them presented themselves at the Alexian Brothers Hospital as agreed.

Upon their arrival at the Chicago hospital Dr Harris informed them he could not permit them to try out the Hoxsey treatment on a patient who had any chance of recovery, but only on a terminal case he had chosen. He, Dr Harris, would watch the patient's reaction, and if the treatment showed any signs of assisting the patient he would turn over more cases who were not so far advanced.

A sixty-six-year-old Sergeant of the Chicago Police Department, Thomas Mannix, was the selected human guinea-pig because he was considered as being incurable. His weight was down to 70 lbs, the pathological report stated he had basal cell carcinoma, and that the malignancy had spread into the clavicular bone of the shoulder. Intensive X-ray therapy had been used, but the disease had not been halted.

Dr Miller was pessimistic with the prognosis. He was sure nothing could help Sergeant Mannix. Hoxsey on the other hand was optimistic. Mrs Stroud, he assured the doctor, had been much worse, yet she had got well.

The treatment started. Within two weeks the surface of the running cancer had begun to dry. A further two weeks later the cancerous mass had begun to shrink, and the patient was able to sit up, had no further need of pain-killing morphine, was eating well, and beginning to gain weight. At the end of six weeks Sergeant Mannix was able to walk, and became impatient to get back to work.

E

In the sixth and seventh week Hoxsey and Miller informed Dr Harris that the time had come to lift out the former cancer growth, and Dr Harris made arrangements for this to be done before members of the hospital medical staff.

It fell to Dr Miller to remove the necrotized mass before about sixty doctors, and in the cavity where the growth had formerly been healthy scar tissue was already forming, and Dr Harris informed his assembled colleagues, 'Gentlemen, you have just witnessed the eighth wonder of the world! We now have a cure for cancer.'

The following morning Dr Harris telephoned Hoxsey asking him to come to his office. According to a record of the meeting Dr Harris told Hoxsey that 'what he had accomplished was the greatest miracle he had ever seen during his entire practice', but warned that they must not let their enthusiasm run away with them. They still had to wait at least five years to make sure there was no recurrence in Sergeant Mannix, and it could not be claimed that the Hoxsey treatment cured cancer until it had been tried out on hundreds of other patients.

What Dr Harris planned was a full-scale, medically controlled trial, if Hoxsey would consent to co-operate. He then put before Harry Hoxsey a ten-page typed document, a contract, which Harris asked Hoxsey to sign before any further steps could be taken.

Hoxsey read through the document very carefully, becoming more and more astonished, as the contract said he must give the Hoxsey herbal formulae to Dr Harris and his associates for a period of ten years. It further stated Hoxsey was to deliver to the doctors ten barrels of the internal medicine, 50 lbs of the powder and 100 lbs of the ointment. Hoxsey was to close his cancer clinic forthwith, and agree not to treat any cases of cancer in future. In return, for the next ten years he was to receive no financial reward, but after that he would get ten per cent of the net profits, while Dr Harris and his colleagues would set the fees to be charged for the treatment and receive 90 per cent of the profits.

Incensed, Hoxsey refused to sign the agreement, and after all attempts at persuasion and threats had failed Dr Harris ripped up the unsigned contract saying, 'If you treat another cancer case we'll send you to jail.'

In addition to that threat Dr Harris contacted the Alexian Brothers Hospital and issued instructions that Harry Hoxsey was not to be allowed to see Sergeant Mannix unless the hospital received prior clearance from him personally.

Faced with the ban the Mannix family was contacted and the Sergeant removed from hospital, and continued to receive the Hoxsey treatment at home for the next six months. After that he was free from cancer. He returned to his job and ten years later died of a heart condition which it was known he already had at the time he was being treated for cancer.

About this case Hoxsey was to write, 'The fact that he died ten years after Dr Malcolm Harris had stated he was incurable and hopeless, and that he died from a heart condition and not of cancer, leads us to believe that the Hoxsey method of treatment is superior to X-ray, radium, and surgery, as this was admittedly a death-bed case. This case is also proof that Dr Harris, as President of the American Medical Association, did everything he could to stop the use of these formulae because he could not control or steal them.'

But despite the threat Hoxsey continued to treat cancer at his clinic in Taylorville, and Dr Harris showed he was not joking as later the same year the official journal of the AMA published the first of many articles branding him as a 'quack', and describing the same treatment which Dr Harris had called the eighth wonder of the world as 'worthless and dangerous to human life'. Doctors working with Hoxsey at the clinic were threatened with the loss of their licence to practise if they continued to associate with Hoxsey, while Hoxsey was arrested four times for practising medicine without a licence; once the Grand Jury refused to indict him on the charge, and three times he had to pay fines of $100.

While all this was happening, on Thursday, 18 July 1929 the town of Girard, Illinois, held a celebration in honour of the Hoxseys and their work with cancer, which was duly reported in the *Girard Gazette* of the time.

Among the people addressing the rally was a Dr Bennett of

Terre Haute, Indiana, who had made a study of the Hoxsey method and then used it in his medical practice. He gave the interesting case history of Mrs Nan Reed, who had a cancer on her eyelid diagnosed at the famous Mayo Institution in Rochester, Minnesota, as epithelioma of the lid. This is what Dr Bennett had to say:

Some 35 years ago there developed a small epithelioma cancer on the upper right eyelid of Mrs Nan Reed of Farmsburg, Indiana. At that time, Aunt Nan, as she was known, went to her family doctor, and he gave her the kindly advice never to bother it until it bothered her.

Later this began to show signs of irritation. She went to one of the noted institutions of the country. It was diagnosed as epithelioma of the lid and treated as such. As time went on this place broke open; she went back and the eye was removed. Later she returned again to this institution, and radium and X-ray were resorted to. The last time she went there they advised her to return home, that all had been done in her case that was to be hoped for.

She returned home and when one of my clinic days came she appeared and was asked into the consulting room. Dr Miller and Dr Hoxsey were there. Aunt Nan seated herself in one of the old-style McDonald chairs. Dr Miller went over in front of her, placed his hands on the arm of the chair, and gazed at her for a while before making the examination, after which he said: 'All of you boys are going to be surprised when I tell you we can cure this case.'

Tears began to roll down the one cheek of Aunt Nan that was left, as one cheek, the entire nose, and one eye were gone, and you could see right back into Aunt Nan's head. There were tears in the eyes of a number of doctors who were in the office at the time, and there were tears streaming down the cheeks of Aunt Nan's son. Aunt Nan was treated that day, and she had quite a reaction because of the amount of tissue involved.

She returned to Farmsburg, and her son stayed with her night and day. Oh, if we had more sons like him! He never left her at any time. When they would ask him to go and get some rest, he would say, 'No, Mother might want something, and I want to be here to serve her to the end.'

I visited her home a number of times, and each time I would remove dead tissue. At the front of the orbit the brain bulged out a half or three-quarters of an inch, protruding right out into the world where it could plainly be seen. At this time we almost gave up hope of saving Aunt Nan, but on account of the nursing and care she got from her son, and with the help of Nature, the hole was filled in, and Aunt Nan is now able to do all her housework again.

This last week Aunt Nan and her son came into my office, and I asked her if she would care if I would call in some doctors to see her case. She said, "Positively not" – as she was glad to let the world see her face and what wonderful results the Hoxsey Method had brought in her case.

So I called in a very prominent eye, ear, nose, and throat specialist who has an office in the same building as me. He came right down. He placed himself directly in front of Aunt Nan and placed his hands in almost the same position that Dr Miller had placed his. He said this was the most remarkable case he had ever seen in his life.

He asked if he could call his partner in to see this case. I said, 'Yes.' He called his partner by phone, but he was busy; he told him regardless of what he was doing at the time to come down to my office, which he did. He called in doctor after doctor, until my office was full of doctors. After taking several looks, each would say to another, 'I wonder what is in Hoxsey's powder?' and 'Dr Bennett, you say you used the powder only one time in this case?'

When I replied, 'Yes,' they said it was surely wonderful.

Since I have been using the Hoxsey Method I have had patients come to me who had been to other physicians, had had their cases diagnosed as cancer, and had been treated by them with X-ray, radium, and surgery – one, two, or all three. To their cases I applied the powder, the cancers dropped out, the wounds healed, and the patients are well again. Ladies and gentlemen, that is why I am using the Hoxsey powder today.

However, popular acclaim of the Girard type did not stop Harry Hoxsey from being hounded by the medical establishment. He was forced to close his Taylorville clinic, and other clinics he established in Iowa, Michigan, West Virginia, New Jersey and Pennsylvania. He finally arrived in Dallas, Texas, in 1936, and from then on until 1950, when he was granted a licence to practise as a Naturopathic Physician – and ND – by the Texas State Board of Examiners, he had more than 100 separate charges of practising medicine without a licence filed against him.

Unlike his father and great-grandfather, Dr Harry Hoxsey did not keep the ingredients of his herbal remedies a secret, nor is the theory underlying the treatment a secret.

Extracts from a treatise written by the former Medical Director of the now defunct Dallas Clinic, Dr J. B. Durkee, shed considerable light on what it was meant to achieve:

Cancer, as you know, can be defined simply as a 'biological process, characterized by a purposeless never-ending cell-division'.

The present treatments of cancer in general acceptance have failed because treatment has been aimed completely at the effects and has ignored the cause. No treatment will ever be successful until physicians and investigators recognize the basic disturbance in body chemistry and cell metabolism. The Hoxsey method of treatment is designed primarily to normalize the body chemistry and control normal cell metabolism.

When a patient enters our clinic, every laboratory procedure is used that might give information as to the patient's general condition, and the extent to which the cancer has progressed. The general classification of cancer as to the various types concerned is of little importance to us in using our treatment. It is important only to prognosis, which we are able to give the patient.

To summarize briefly, we have a successful treatment of cancer, as proven by hundreds of cured patients. We have proof that cancer has one basic cause, regardless of the classification. Third, because we know that our medication changes the blood chemistry, we have the reasonable belief that the cause of cancer is to be found in a disturbance of the inorganic and organic chemistry of the blood-stream and tissue fluids.

Therefore, we strongly recommend intensive, widespread, and continuing research along these lines, coupled with the widest possible exchange of information and theory. If this is done, it will not be long before the basic cause of cancer is proven conclusively, and increasingly effective methods of treatment introduced into common usage. We are already conquering cancer; it will not be long before that conquest is complete.[3]

Dr Hoxsey described his treatment as chemotherapy, and said:

We consider cancer a systemic disease. We are convinced that, without exception, it occurs only in the presence of profound physiological change in the constituents of body fluids and a consequent chemical imbalance in the organism. This concept, based on extensive practical experience in treating thousands of cancer cases, is in full accord with the most advanced research by specialists, who admit the futility of approaching the problem with surgery, radium and X-ray[4]

What Doctors Durkee and Hoxsey failed to mention in their explanations or theories of cancer is *why* the profound physiological changes occur. A possible answer was expounded by Dr Gotthard Booth of New York City in various papers he has written to the effect that the origins of cancer are to be found in the mental state of the patient, and that cancer is a psychosomatic condition in which the mind triggers off physiological changes.[5]

After all this, and to help the reader reach a personal decision as to whether herbs can cure cancer, there is a statement appearing in the handbook, the 'March of Truth on Cancer',[6] made by its compiler, Mr Arlin J. Brown: 'Estimates of the number of cancer patients cured by the Hoxsey cancer method range from 25,000 to 75,000. In fact, a certain US Congressman discouraged Dr Hoxsey from carrying out a plan to have 25,000 of his cured patients picket the White House.' That sounds impressive, but to counterbalance it the American Medical Association asserts that the herbal formulae formerly used by Harry Hoxsey are 'worthless' and little more than 'cough-mixture'. As I have been unable to find any records of the Hoxsey method ever being submitted to a full medically controlled test by any of the leading cancer research groups in the United States or elsewhere, I mentioned to a prominent British researcher into cancer – a member of the orthodoxy rather than the heterodoxy – that I intended to write a chapter about the possible use of herbs in the war against cancer. I was told, 'Yes, I'm sure there are certain herbs which can cure certain types of cancer.' I was pleased to hear the comment, and enquired if I could quote the doctor by name, only to hear the words, 'Don't be silly!'

6

Profession First –
Patients Second?

It would seem to be beyond the realm of credibility to imagine a situation where a drugless practitioner using herbal remedies may have discovered a cure for some internal and many external cancers which do not respond to current orthodox treatment, and instead of being hailed as a benefactor to mankind has become the victim of a conspiracy to silence him; a conspiracy to prevent his alleged 'cure' from being fully investigated to ascertain whether the claims made for it were genuine; to prevent him from treating even those people who had been condemned to death by acknowledged orthodox cancer specialists; and finally to prevent him from writing about or sending any details of his work through the mails to those interested in learning more about what he had done in the past and what may be possible in the future.

Incredible though such a situation would be, from the available evidence it appears this may have already happened in the United States. What makes the case more alarming, if that were possible, is a statement made in a court of law by a lawyer acting for the Texas State Board of Medical Examiners, the latter being the official medical body in the State of Texas which licenses doctors to practise within the State.

In May 1956, the lawyer in question, a Mr Julian C. Hyer, asked that the charge against Harry Hoxsey and the officially licensed doctors working with him, to the effect that the treatment then being used at the Hoxsey Cancer Clinic in Dallas was worthless, be stricken from the record of the case, and during the legal arguments that ensued Mr Hyer said, *'We don't deny that they cure cancer out there at the clinic.'*

That amazing admission, qualified by medical pundits to mean they recognize Hoxsey was able to cure certain *external* cancers as opposed to internal malignancies, was made at a point in a legal case where Harry Hoxsey brought a group of his former patients into the courtroom – among them being a Dr H. K. Hill, MD, of Laverne, Oklahoma – and his lawyers were ready to put each one separately into the witness box to prove, by presenting biopsy, hospital and clinical records, etc., that all of them had previously proven cancers, both internal and external, but had been cured by the Hoxsey treatment. Rather than have a procession of former cancer victims testify to that effect the legal spokesman for orthodox medicine in the State of Texas was prepared to admit that the Hoxsey Clinic was curing cancer.

If the acknowledgement was insufficient to prompt a full investigation of the Hoxsey treatment to appraise its efficacy, there were other equally important developments which should have made it imperative.

Two years before Mr Hyer's statement a group of ten doctors from all parts of the United States, some of them with a wide experience of cancer, assembled at the Hoxsey Clinic to examine what was really happening there. They had no official standing other than being qualified and licensed to practise medicine in their respective States, and their only common interest was to try and ascertain the truth.

This medical group examined the backgrounds of the staff at the clinic, and the facilities, to see if they were adequate, and with Dr E. E. Loffler, MD, of Spokane, Washington, acting as the chairman, investigated more than a score of former Hoxsey patient case histories, and then questioned the patients thoroughly.

At the end of the investigatory period the doctors released a report confirming that the facilities and staff were above reproach, and:

. . . This Clinic now has under treatment or observation

between four and five thousand cancer patients. It handles approximately ninety patients per day. Approximately 100 new patients per week come to the Clinic seeking relief, and the evidence we have seen indicates that approximately 90 per cent of these are terminal cases. Over the years the Clinic has accumulated more than 10,000 case histories, photographic studies and X-ray studies of patients from all over the United States, Canada, Alaska, Mexico, Hawaii, the Canal Zone and elsewhere.[1]

We find as a fact that our investigation has demonstrated to our satisfaction that the Hoxsey Cancer Clinic in Dallas, Texas, is successfully treating pathologically proven cases of cancer, both internal and external, without the use of surgery, radium or X-ray.[2]

Accepting the standard yardstick of cases that have remained symptom-free in excess of five or six years after treatment, established by medical authorities, we have seen sufficient cases to warrant such a conclusion. Some of those presented before us have been free of symptoms as long as twenty-four years, and the physical evidence indicates that they are all enjoying exceptional health at this time.

We, as a Committee feel that the Hoxsey treatment is superior to such conventional methods of treatment as X-ray, radium and surgery. We are willing to assist this Clinic in any way possible in bringing this treatment to the American public. We are willing to use it in our office, in our practice on our own patients when, at our discretion, it is deemed necessary.

The above statement represents the unanimous findings of this Committee. In testimony thereof we hereby attach our signatures.[3]

Among the former Hoxsey patients appearing before the *ad hoc* committee was Dr H. K. Hill, MD, who testified he had developed a cancer in his lower, left side, and before he went to the Clinic it had started oozing matter which had a putrid smell. He gave the names of three surgeons who had confirmed the diagnosis as malignant carcinoma, and told the members of the committee, 'They offered to remove the growth for me several times, free of charge, but I could not bring myself to submit. I preferred to wait. I did not want surgical treatment.'

When asked why he did not agree to undergo surgery Dr Hill replied that he had known someone who had had the same type of cancer as himself surgically removed, but it did not help and the man died. He admitted that after being a doctor for thirty-one years many of his colleagues had criticized his decision to seek treatment at the Dallas Clinic, but in answer to the question, 'Do you consider that the cancer is absorbed?' his answer was, 'Yes, in fact it is completely healed.'

Another person who testified was a former Olympic wrestling champion, Joe Parelli, who in 1947 was diagnosed as having cancer of the left jaw, and after having part of the bone removed was finally hospitalized. His condition continued to deteriorate while he was in hospital and a priest was sent for to administer the last sacrament as his death seemed imminent. It was then, when it appeared his last hour on earth was approaching, a group of his friends took him to the Hoxsey Clinic.

The examining panel of doctors asked Mr Parelli what had happening after he commenced the Hoxsey treatment.

'I started to get well. They gave me medicine and I started feeling good. Then they put some powder and salve on my cancer. I started gaining weight, gaining strength, and I could eat. The other doctors used to feed me with a needle in the vein, but after coming here I started eating normal.'

He was asked to continue with his story.

'In three months the bone cancer came out. Nobody picked it out. It just fell out. That's what the Hoxsey treatment did for me. It cured me. Today I am as strong as a bull.'

Seen overall it was a remarkable document. It gave a positive conclusion, while at the same time it countered two of the main objections that orthodox medicine usually raises whenever a heterodox therapy is quoted as having some success with cancer, namely that there could have been a wrong diagnosis or the cure could have occurred without any treatment through spontaneous remission.

Another reason why the report should not have been dismissed is that all the men comprising the examining body were originally hostile to Hoxsey and only went to Dallas after a Pennsylvania State Senator, John J. Haluska, had launched a newspaper campaign telling the readers of his column in the local press what Hoxsey was achieving.

Just how Senator Haluska came into the picture makes interesting reading.

Back in the 1940s the Senator's eight-year-old son had died after being operated upon for cancer, and some years later, while he was working as a Hospital Administrator at the Miners Hospital in Spangler, Pa., his family doctor walked into his office and informed him that his younger sister, Mrs Verne Kielbowick, had also got cancer and was doomed to die. The doctor explained the malignancy had started in the cervix but had become metastasized throughout the entire body. 'We have taken biopsy after biopsy to make certain we are right,' he said, 'because we know how close she is to you. We have no answer.'

Following their conversation Mrs Kielbowick was taken to Pittsburg by ambulance for an operation. It was a wasted journey. After making an incision she was immediately sewn up again as there was nothing that could be done. The specialist explained, 'She is rotten inside. We will give her morphine and let her die a painless death.'

The Senator was unable to accept that. He had previously heard stories about Hoxsey, most of them derogatory, and was dubious to say the least, but when he realized orthodox medicine had nothing more to offer his sister he threw caution to the wind and telephoned Harry Hoxsey in Dallas. He read the pathology report signed by Dr Brumbaugh, and Hoxsey's reaction was, 'Senator, I am not God. I cannot do the impossible. I am only human, but I have cured thousands of people. Unfortunately, they come here when they are ready to take their last breath. I figure you will save yourself money to follow the doctor's advise and let her die a natural death.'

That advice was equally unacceptable, and he asked Hoxsey to take his sister as a patient, explaining that if she died on the journey to Texas no one would hold him responsible.

Mrs Kielbowick made the trip and her cancer remissed.

Once she was well again Senator Haluska wrote about what

had happened in his local newspaper. There was an immediate and favourable response from the local County Medical Society, and a newspaper headline read, 'Cambria Medical Society Back Senator Haluska's Stand'.

Two hundred doctors held a meeting to discuss the developments then sent a letter to US Senator Langer explaining how, apparently, an important medical discovery had been made. They asked him to investigate the treatment, and if what Haluska said was proven to be correct they wanted it to be introduced into every hospital throughout the nation.

Three days after the local medical society's meeting a representative of the national American Medical Association arrived upon the scene and demanded to know who had given them permission to call such a meeting, and why they had asked for an investigation. 'Don't you men know that Hoxsey is the greatest enemy we have?' the spokesman for the AMA is quoted as saying. 'We have had him in court now for a quarter of a century, time in and time out. He is a charlatan; he is a quack. Give that man a chance and he will spread throughout the country. He will do us harm. Now, we know that you cannot back down politely, but from now on keep quiet.'

The local doctors took the hint, and while Haluska kept on pressing them to make their own investigation, even suggesting he would personally pay all expenses for a committee to go to Dallas and examine the evidence, they refused.

He continued to publicize Hoxsey until one day he received from Dr H. B. Mueller, MD, of Cleveland, Ohio, an Instructor of Internal Medicine at the University of Michigan, a letter in which Dr Mueller attacked Haluska for keeping up his newspaper campaign. 'We have taken all the abuse we are going to take from you cheap politicians back there in Pennsylvania . . .' he wrote, and informed the Senator that seven doctors were going to Dallas in April 1954, adding, 'we want you to be there and be sure you are there.'

While Senator and Mrs Haluska were making arrangements to be in Dallas at the specified time they got a surprise. The Cambria County Medical Society informed them it was sending a chief surgeon, Dr Benjamin F. Bowers of Evansburg, Pa., together with a newspaper reporter, a Mr McDevitt, and made the comment, 'We shall see what this man Hoxsey has.'

At the clinic the seven doctors refused to shake hands with 'the cheap politician', but Hoxsey gave them thirty-five proven cases of internal and external cancer in both men and women to examine. Not content with merely placing his records before the seven doctors, Hoxsey sent telegrams to Dr J. R. Heller of the National Cancer Institute in Maryland, to John Teeter of the Damon Runyon Cancer Fund of New York, to Dr Cameron, Medical Director of the American Cancer Society; to Dr Leonard Sheele, the US Surgeon General, and Oliver Field, the lawyer for the American Medical Association, which read:

> Thirty-five pathological proven cases of cures, internal and external, of cancer will be presented before a jury of seven MDs from all over the Nation at the Hoxsey Cancer Clinic, Dallas, Texas, April 10, 11, 12, 1954. You are invited to attend or send representatives. (signed) Dr Harry M. Hoxsey.

By the appointed date three more doctors, none of them representing the organizations the telegrams had been sent to, arrived to swell the medical panel to ten. They carried out their investigation, and these formerly antagonistic medical men issued their statement that Hoxsey was curing both internal and external cancer.[4]

Yet the report had little effect, and was soon pushed well under a blanket of silence. In this respect it was history repeating itself, for long prior to its release Harry Hoxsey and a number of US Senators had repeatedly asked for a full investigation. Hoxsey had given written guarantees that in the event his remedies were found to be worthless he would donate $25,000 to any named charity and then close the doors of his clinic once and for all. But nothing was ever done and the details behind organized medicine's, 'don't confuse us with the facts, because they simply don't fit into current medical thinking,' reads more like a thriller-novel of Nazi repression as every attempt to get an exhaustive clinical study made was dictatorially suppressed, and the public deliberately brainwashed by a barrage of misleading propaganda.

As this is a serious accusation to make against the American allopathic medical hierarchy, which claims to have the best interests of patients at heart, it cannot remain without substantiation. What happened to the efforts made by the late US Senator Charles Tobey of New Hampshire will more than suffice in doing this.

Senator Tobey became interested in the numerous heterodox methods of treating cancer after his son, Charles Tobey, Jr, was striken with incurable cancer, the diagnosis being confirmed at Tufts Medical School and at Columbia University College of Physicians and Surgeons. Charles Tobey then underwent a remission after Dr Robert E. Lincoln of Bedford, Mass., treated him with his own therapeutic discovery, bacteriophage. His father tried to get the Senate to launch a full-scale investigation into finding how effective non-recognized cancer treatments were, only to find he kept on running into an invisible wall. His every attempt was blocked. Then, early in 1953, Senator Tobey became chairman of the Senate Interstate Commerce Committee, and he thought up a stratagem which would breach the barriers of obstruction he had met previously. Without telling his colleagues on the Committee he decided to assemble an investigatory staff whose sole term of reference would be to conduct a secret, preliminary survey of the heterodox cancer situation, paying particular attention to 'the alleged interstate conspiracy engaged in by individuals and combines of any kind whatsoever to hinder, suppress or restrict the free flow of drugs, research and methods relating to the cause, prevention and systems of diagnosis and treatment' of cancer.

Needing a trained investigator to head the new team the Senator approached his friend, the then US Attorney General, Herbert Brownell, who recommended a thirty-five-year-old lawyer, Mr Benedict F. FitzGerald, Jr, currently working as a trial lawyer for the Department of Justice; a man who had previously been a lawyer for the National Labour Relations Board, and a legal counsel to a Congressional Committee.

After winding up the work he was doing Mr FitzGerald spent six months looking into heterodox methods of treating cancer and the opposition to such methods, but a few weeks before he submitted his preliminary report to Senator Tobey, fate stepped in. The seventy-three-year-old Senator died and was succeeded as chairman by Senator Bricker of Ohio.

In the FitzGerald Report which was filed with the Committee on 11 August 1953, and became a part of the Congressional Record on 28 August 1953,[5] the investigator wrote:

The attention of the Committee is invited to the request made by Senator Elmer Thomas following an investigation made by the Senator of the Hoxsey Cancer Clinic under the date of February 25th, 1947, and addressed to the Surgeon General, Public Health Department, Washington, DC, wherein he sought to enlist the support of the Federal Government to make an investigation and report. No such investigation was made. In fact, every effort was made to avoid and evade the investigation by the Surgeon General's office. The record will reveal that this clinic did furnish sixty-two complete case histories, including pathology, names of hospitals, physicians, etc., in 1945. Again in June 1950, seventy-seven case histories, which included the names of the patients, pathological reports in many instances, and in the absence thereof, the names of the pathologists, hospitals and physicians who had treated these patients before being treated at the Hoxsey Cancer Clinic. The Council of National Cancer Institute, without investigation, in October, 1950, refused to order an investigation. The record in the Federal Court discloses that this agency of the Federal Government took sides and sought in every way to hinder, suppress and restrict this institution in their treatment of cancer ...

At another place in his report Mr FitzGerald gave his assessment of the machinations surrounding another heterodox cancer therapy, Krebiozen:

The controversy is involved and requires further research and development. There is reason to believe that the AMA [American Medical Association] has been hasty, capricious, arbitrary, and downright dishonest, and of course if the doctrine of 'respondeat superior' is to be observed, the alleged machinations of Dr J. J. Moore [for the past ten years

F   81 treasurer of the AMA] could involve the AMA and others in interstate conspiracy of alarming proportions . . .[6]

These two short extracts from the seventeen page document show it was political dynamite, and the new chairman of the Interstate Commerce Committee, Senator Bricker, wanted no part of it. He refused to see Mr FitzGerald to discuss his findings even when FitzGerald offered to fly out to Ohio at his own expense for an interview, and a member of the Senator's office advised the investigator that the best thing for all concerned was to forget about the whole affair and, above all, not to talk to the press. A promise was then made that if FitzGerald did what was asked he would be 'taken care of'.

Shaken by the reaction FitzGerald wrote to Senator Bricker that he 'was surprised and even shocked' at what was happening to him. But his protest got him nowhere. His position with the Committee was abruptly terminated, and when he returned to the Department of Justice, where he had previously worked and from where he was 'on loan', he discovered he did not work there either.

The next step in this tale of intrigue and skulduggery was that Senator Bricker side-stepped the issue by announcing that his Committee lacked the jurisdiction to investigate cancer, and he suggested that if an alleged conspiracy was involved this would be a matter for the Senate Judiciary Committee under the chairmanship of Senator William E. Langer.

FitzGerald realized the buck had been passed to Senator Langer and on 21 September 1953 wrote him a devastating precis of his findings.

Mentioning his earlier report and his recommendation Fitz-Gerald wrote:

> I would like to make it again—that the United States Senate should take jurisdiction of this problem and formally determine whether existing agencies, both public and private, have engaged in and pursued a policy of harassment, ridicule, slander and libellous attacks on those who appear to be sincerely engaged in stamping out this curse of mankind – the dreaded disease cancer.

My investigation of this subject indicates that there is evidence that organized medicine, working through medical associations, has engaged in this practice to such an extent that their efforts amount to a giant conspiracy . . .

About Harry M. Hoxsey he wrote in his letter to Senator Langer:

For over a quarter of a century it appears there has been some speculation over the therapeutic value of the Hoxsey method of curing cancer, with many champions representing both sides. I know that you attempted to face this problem several times before and that you visited the Hoxsey Clinic in Dallas, Texas, yourself in 1951 and during the same year in the 82nd Congress you deemed it necessary to propose a Senate investigation of the matter, but for some reason your efforts were thwarted.

The Senate Bill introduced by Senator Langer was not accepted although at the time of visiting the Clinic a Dallas newspaper quoted him as saying, 'If Hoxsey can cure eighty per cent of his cases, then the American public is entitled to that knowledge. If, on the other hand, the Clinic can't cure cancer, then the public is entitled to know that too.'

However, to continue with the FitzGerald letter:

At this point, I wish to make my position clear: I am a lawyer, not a doctor, and I do not wish to assume the task of appraising the therapeutic value of any particular method of treating cancer, especially where there is conflict between medical men. I feel obliged to report to you, however, that with respect to the legality of the actions waged against the Hoxsey method, they constitute a legal invasion of his personal liberties and they amount to a conspiracy.

From the evidence I have gathered, it appears that as early as 1924 the Hoxsey method of treating cancer was considered so effective by a former president of the medical association that he personally presented its sponsor with a written proposal which, among other things, provided for the relinquishment

of valuable property rights in the Hoxsey method and medicines and formulae to this same official.

The evidence indicates that when the proposition was
spurned, Hoxsey was advised to sign and accept the proposal
or face ruination. Such tactics, if true, constitute blackmail of
the rankest order and this evidence should be examined closely
to ascertain its credulity.

During the years that followed there is evidence that
Hoxsey, in attempting to present his methods of treating
cancer to the American public, rapidly became the target of a
most vituperative type of activity that could possibly be
bestowed upon any living individual. Attempts on his part to
assist in the administration of the Hoxsey method were frus-
trated from every angle, and he was frequently thrown in
jail . . . On each occasion there is evidence that medical associations, throughout the country, operating under orders from
headquarters in Chicago, brought about his arrest and initiated
filing of complaints against him at virtually every turn.

In all but three instances, where criminal actions were instituted, the evidence shows that the defendant was acquitted,
and on the three occasions during which convictions were
entered, Hoxsey alleges that a plea of guilty was entered for
the purpose of saving time and money. Throughout the entire
period he was continually required to retain counsel and defend
himself from charges which were constantly emanating from
the same source . . .

The evidence further shows that on 18 March 1949, Hoxsey
brought suit for libel and slander against Dr Morris Fishbein,
who at that time was Editor of the American Medical Association Journal, and after three years of legal manoeuvring, Dr
Fishbein was found guilty, in the District Court, 44th Judicial
District in Dallas County, Texas.

The technique employed by the medical associations in
harassing and libelling was clearly pointed out in this trial.
The evidence reveals organized medicine instituted the preparation of scurrilous articles on 2 January 1926, 3 August
1929 and 19 March 1932 and caused them to be inserted in
medical journals and newspapers throughout the country . . .

This was followed by the circulation of reprints and photo-stats of the 'poisoned pen' variety to individuals throughout the entire nation in a carefully planned and concerted attempt, calculated to destroy the Hoxsey method of treating cancer . . .

Meanwhile the office of the American Cancer Society and the Surgeon General of the United States Army were also deluged with copies of scurrilous articles and they in turn would distribute the material without further investigation to all who made inquiry concerning the Hoxsey method of treatment . . .

During the period of approximately a quarter of a century, there is evidence of a continuous attempt to hinder, suppress and restrict the activity of licensed practitioners who attempted to associate themselves with Hoxsey and his methods.

The technique in these instances included the summoning of medical practitioners before local medical boards and upon their appearance each was threatened to refrain from associating with Hoxsey and his methods or face the possibilities of a revocation of their license.

Such was the situation with respect to the treatment of Dr C. M. Hartzog of Gulfport, Mississippi whose testimony in this regard is set forth in a deposition taken on 23 May 1952 in connection with the case of Harry M. Hoxsey vs Morris Fishbein in the 44th District Court, Dallas, Texas . . .

Mr FitzGerald next listed by name and town twenty-two doctors from ten States who were threatened by their local medical associations for supporting the use of the Hoxsey treatment in certain selected cases.

Thus the conspiracy continued and on 2 February 1947 its extensiveness was publicly noted by the Honorable Elmer Thomas, at that time United States Senator from Oklahoma who wrote:

It seems that the medical fraternity is highly organized and that they decided to crush you and your institution, if at all possible. I have had a few 'rounds' with the heads of the medical organization as well as the Public Health Service here in Washington and it seems that the public officials are afraid that if they make any move, or say anything antagonistic to the wishes of the medical organization that they will be pounced upon and destroyed. In other words, the public officials seem afraid of their jobs and even of their lives. This presents a most serious case and I am at a loss to know how to proceed.

The history of organized medicine throughout America differs greatly from the history of organized medicine in other civilized areas. In our great country medical associations have been infected with intrigue, discrimination and collusion. Not long ago this culminated in Federal convictions which found violations of the Sherman Anti-Trust Law.

In gathering information in connection with my study, I have not abandoned my general esteem for the great majority of the men engaged in the medical profession throughout America. I have continued to retain a high respect for those who conscientiously heal the sick and endeavour to alleviate pain.

However, I have hesitated to accept the philosophy of the medical associations, which would inject a philosophy of tyranny by attempting to annihilate the basic concepts of American liberty by discrimination against professional men merely because of their particular medical classification.

The law in many jurisdictions has attached a certain dignity to the several branches of the profession and the Osteopathic Physician and Surgeon, the Naturopathic Physician, and the Chiropractor are all entitled to its protection, regardless of their lack of membership in a particular assocation.

I have pointed out this involvement of organized medicine with respect to the hindrance and the free flow of drugs and the harassment of our citizens. These situations amount to a CONSPIRACY and that should warrant your Committee in taking jurisdiction and conducting an immediate investigation for the expressed purpose of gathering the facts and drafting protective legislation.

The fact that various agencies of the Federal Government are manned by officials who are also active in medical associations requires a consideration as to whether or not these officials are directing their first allegiance to the citizens and government of America – or to these same medical associations. I shall look forward to and appreciate your serious consideration of this grave problem.

Respectfully yours,

(signed) Benedict F. FitzGerald, Jr

Again these efforts to arrive at the truth were fruitless, and it was not too surprising because in addition to active opposition from the powerful American Medical Association, Hoxsey and others in the field of non-recognized cancer treatments had to contend with opposition from a Federal agency, the Food and Drug Administration (FDA).

As far as I have been able to ascertain the FDA first took concrete action against Hoxsey in 1950 when it instigated a court action to prevent him from sending his medications through the mails and into Interstate Commerce.

After hearing testimony from a number of patients apparently cured of cancer at the Dallas Clinic the presiding judge, following the jury's verdict which went against the FDA, stated, 'That the respondent's treatment is not injurious. Some it cures, and some it does not cure, and some it relieves somewhat.'

Of course the FDA could not take that defeat lying down, and it appealed the verdict to the Fifth Court of Appeals at New Orleans where it obtained a reversal of the lower Court's decision in a manner which many people who have made a study of the legal aspects of this entire affair maintain was highly suspect.

Yet, it was in 1955–6 that the FDA resorted to tactics which should be subjected to a separate investigation because its officers appear to have resorted to deliberate lying to smear the Hoxsey method.

In 1955 Senator Haluska opened a Hoxsey Clinic at Portage, Pennsylvania, under the medical direction of Dr Newton C. Allen, DO, an osteopathic physician who also held a Doctorate in Medicine, an MD.

Soon after the Portage Clinic opened its doors, an officer of the Food and Drug Administration made his appearance and made certain demands upon Dr Allen which the latter considered to be contrary to the law of the land, and further, if he complied with the demands, he considered he would be breaching his professional patient-practitioner relationship. Dr Allen therefore refused to do what he was asked. Upon hearing his refusal the FDA officer promised the doctor that his lack of co-operation would result in his being prevented from continuing the practice of medicine.

It was not an idle threat for shortly afterwards an announcement was made to the press from the office of the US Attorney in Pittsburg to the effect that the Government would commence action against Dr Allen; that Dr Allen was a quack; that the Government would interrogate his patients and seize any medications, and Dr Allen would be charged with numerous criminal and civil violations of the law.

On 1 April 1955, officers of the law arrested Dr Allen, charging him with criminal violations of the medical practices act of the Commonwealth of Pennsylvania, namely of not being a physician, and practising medicine without a licence.

Dr Allen asked the officers to look at his credentials which were hanging upon the wall of his office, showing conclusively that he was a properly licensed physician in the State of Pennsylvania, and was also licensed to practice medicine in several other States as well. He pointed to his MD degree, and suggested to the officers there must have been a mistake. The officers ignored his protestations, and the doctor was faced with posting a bail-bond or remaining in jail until his trial.

Newspapers, radio and television gave this news item, of Dr Allen's arrest, the headline treatment while government officials continued to hold 'private' press-conferences where newsmen were given lurid and incorrect information as a part of the smear campaign.

Dr Allen remained branded a 'quack' until Thursday, 15 December 1955 – some nine months – when the District Attorney for Washington County, Pa., Mr Ray Zelt, appeared in court before Judge David Weiner and informed the court, among other things, 'that Dr Newton C. Allen was a properly registered Osteopathic Physician and in addition thereto held an MD degree . . .' and 'that actually no person or persons were prepared to go into court to sue Dr Allen . . .' Mr Zelt accordingly entered a plea of 'nolle pros.' – unwillingness to prosecute.

The judge accepted the District Attorney's statement and all charges against Dr Allen were razed from the records. But, what is interesting is that none of the government officials, nor spokesmen for the FDA who had called Dr Allen a charlatan and a quack were prepared to go into court and put themselves in the witness box and under oath!

Nor was the FDA's actions in the subsequent chapters of the Hoxsey saga free from criticism, yet in the end the combined forces of the AMA and FDA won, and today the Hoxsey treatment as far as the US is concerned has been relegated to the trash can.

To me this all smacks of professionalism taking precedence over the welfare of patients: it would have been much easier and more scientific if the AMA and FDA had run clinical trials as the former president of the AMA, Dr Harris, had suggested. Then the public would have known the facts and been able to decide for themselves whether the Hoxsey therapy was a hoax or a real glimpse of hope.

But, if the reader thinks that what I have written above could only happen in the United States of America and nowhere else they would be mistaken. In Europe there have been numerous cases of allopathically trained, orthodox doctors who, after using heterodox methods of treating cancer, have found themselves hauled into court charged with manslaughter, and have been victims of conspiracies instigated by their medical associations. A prime example is the case of the controversial German physician, Dr Josef Issels. Anyone reading his biography *Issels: The Biography of a Doctor* by Gordon Thomas[7] – will see how organized medicine was prepared to go to any lengths to destroy him; something it has now achieved as he has been forced to close his clinic. And the machinations of various British doctors in trying to prevent the British Broadcasting Corporation from televizing the Issels documentary film *Go Climb a Mountain,* plus the pressure put upon a prominent medical researcher to make him cease researching into the efficacy of the Issels treatment leave a very unpleasant taste lingering in the mouth.

Why does it happen?

A possible explanation appeared in the US magazine *Saturday Evening Post,* dated 21 December 1946, when it stated, 'A doctor who claims to know an effective treatment for cancer not involving surgery, radium or X-ray is an *ipso facto* quack.'

However, the British are fortunate, for the type of trial by news-media indulged in by certain senior US officials during the Hoxsey 'Pittsburg Trial' of 1956 could not happen here. On the contrary, although the General Medical Council forbids a registered medical practitioner from passing on a patient to an unregistered practitioner, when the Foster Commission investigating Scientology recommended limiting the activities of lay-psychotherapists, the British Medical Association came out against the recommendation.

Sir Ronald Tunbridge, chairman of the BMA's Board of Science and Education said that while there were obvious dangers, he recognized that the lay-psychotherapists had been responsible for some new ideas. 'We are not wishing to be exclusive. We don't think we know all the answers,' Sir Ronald told a reporter from *The Daily Telegraph.*[8]

The open-minded attitude of the British Medical Association is reminiscent of that of the famous scientist Alexis Carrel:

> More than half the great remedies known to medical history have come from empiricists; this is from 'irregulars', men and women of no or little scientific training. There is no reason to believe that conditions have essentially changed. In the future an unregistered, self-trained experimenter, an 'empiricist' by strict classification, may just as well make a revolutionary medical discovery as one employed in a great laboratory having every up-to-date equipment.

Was Harry M. Hoxsey, I wonder, one of Carrel's empiricists?

7

A Little Does You More Good – Homeopathy

The disquiet about the orthodox medical profession's use of large and persistent doses of toxic drugs is not a recent phenomenon. For as far back as the end of the eighteenth century a German doctor, Samuel Hahnemann, was appalled and sadly disillusioned at what his medical colleagues were doing with crude drug therapy which he felt did more harm than good; and it was these conclusions which led him to look for an alternative system of medicine that would be safe, gentle and effective.

Hahnemann also differed from other medical practitioners since he believed that in everyone there was a natural healing capacity, and that if anybody became ill the symptoms which appeared were not in themselves the illness, but were the outward, visible signs of the body's fight against the disease. Therefore, he postulated, it was the physician's duty to assist the healing forces of nature by carefully noting how the body fought disease, by studying the symptoms, and when that had been concluded to administer a drug that would reproduce identical physical reactions in a healthy person.

The concept that drugs are meant to suppress all the outward signs of sickness, and that once the symptoms have disappeared the patient can be considered as 'cured', is still current, orthodox medical thought that is drilled into medical students as they go through their years of study in medical school. As a result of this reasoning when a patient with a high temperature goes to see his doctor a medicine is prescribed to lower it, and when the temperature becomes normal it is assumed the patient is well again. But, does the remission of the symptom, in this case the high temperature, mean the person is cured of what originally caused the fever? Or does the suppressed cause continue to lurk inside the body waiting to reappear when another illness strikes, making the next 'cure' more difficult to achieve?

Partial evidence to show this may well happen was given to me by a leading British naturopathic and osteopathic practitioner, Mr Sidney Rose-Neil, when we were discussing how patients undergoing naturopathic treatment regress back through previously suppressed illnesses before they achieve good health.

When we put our patients on to a fast, and then an individually prepared diet, they often do regress. They regress backwards through illnesses they have had, right through childhood, and although the reappearance of the symptoms is not as prolonged as the original sickness, the symptoms are there and recognizable. If you have not got a full case history, and this happens, it can be alarming when you see the symptoms, because in some cases they are severe.

For instance, if a person has had scarlet fever as a child, their body can throw up all the physical signs of scarlet fever. Fortunately the naturopath has been taught to expect this regression to happen occasionally, and it is after their regression that we consider the body is ready to start functioning properly . . .[1]

Mr Rose-Neil's comment could be dismissed as biased because he is a drugless therapist with an axe to grind. However, the same could not be said of Berton Roueché when, in his book *The Incurable Wound*,[2] about the side-effects of artificially produced cortisone, he said, 'It has the power to revive a vanquished infection, it can excite a latent one to manifest itself and, in the opinion of some investigators, it may even be capable of transforming into antagonists certain normally innocuous viruses . . .'

More on the same theme is to be found in the book *Medicine – Rational and Irrational* by Cyril Scott,[3] in which he describes how a 27-year-old woman was found to have diabetes and immediately placed upon a strict diet, was given insulin, and had regular urine checks for sugar. In spite of the treatment her condition deteriorated and blood transfusions became necessary. She implored her doctors to cease the insulin injections because they made her feel worse. Her pleas were ignored. It was then she was taken to see Mr Ellis Barker, who wasn't too interested in her diabetes – the presenting symptom – but very interested in trying to discover the underlying cause. His search was not in vain. He found she had had measles when she was seven years old, and although she appeared to have been cured, the measles had only been suppressed. Mr Barker gave the patient a homeopathic dose of morbillinum, and she developed a measles rash over the entire body area, a phenomenon which Cyril Scott wrote was 'Nature's method of getting rid of the poisons'. When the rash subsided she began to get well. Mr Barker ordered that she have massage, eat a lot of bran in increasing quantities, and at the same time reduce the insulin down to zero – something she was able to do within a fortnight. Over the next two years, when this lady's case history was written up, there were no signs of her diabetes, and she found she was able to eat foodstuffs formerly forbidden her by orthodox practitioners.

Just how Dr Hahnemann rediscovered the principle that 'like cures like' occurred in 1790 when he was translating a *Materia Medica* written by an Englishman called Cullen. He read what Cullen said about the curative value of Peruvian Bark in the treatment of fevers, and was critical of the claims made for it. As a scientist with doubts he decided to test Peruvian Bark on himself to see what the effect was. 'I took for several days four drachms of good cinchona twice daily', and he discovered the symptoms it gave him 'were those which to me are typical of intermittent fevers.' He carried on with further experimentation and arrived at the conclusion: 'It is only by the power to make sick that drugs can cure sickness: and that a medicine can only cure such morbid conditions as it can produce, when tested on healthy persons.'

Unlike many others Hahnemann did not immediately publish his findings. Instead he spent the next six years experimenting and observing the effects of drugs on healthy people, effects which he referred to as being a 'symptom picture'. And only when he was sure he was on the right track towards a safer system of medicine did he write his 'Essay on the New Principle', which was published in 1796 in *Hufeland's Journal*.

It was during the six years of experimentation that he discovered the dosage of the drug was immaterial, and a small amount of a drug worked as effectively as a larger one. This part of his research was as important then as it is today as an alternative to the over-prescribing of drugs, but it led to increasing antagonism both from the ranks of the medical profession, who saw his work as heresy, and from the apothecaries – the chemists – who saw his minute drug doses as being a way of undermining their livelihood.

At that time in Leipsic there was a law on the statute books which forbade anyone other than apothecaries from mixing medicines, and prevented any doctor from giving a medicine directly to a patient. The druggists reported Hahnemann to the town council for breaking both of the laws. Dr Hahnemann was duly brought into court on 15 March 1820, and ordered to refrain from his activities. The decision was a severe blow to him as the laws used to limit this practice were never meant to cover the particular situation which homeopathy presented. Yet he eventually overcame the problem as a few apothecaries agreed to make up his homeopathic remedies.

On the purely medical side, the attack against him manifested itself in Leipsic University, where the medical students who attended Hahnemann's classes were penalized for refusing to dissociate themselves from homeopathy. In certain instances Dr Clarus, the Clinical Professor at the University and the foremost medical authority in Saxony, refused to pass medical students whom he felt were too closely involved in Hahnemann's work.

In 1831 cholera swept through Europe and Hahnemann set out to find a cure based upon his method of 'provings' – to find a substance which would bring about the symptoms of cholera in healthy people; and he discovered that camphor gave the same 'symptom picture', although later he used copper and other remedies.

He wrote up his findings on camphor and arranged for leaflets to be printed and circulated to doctors in the worst-afflicted areas, in order that they might have in their hands a weapon to combat the epidemic. But his adversary Dr Clarus at Leipsic University did everything possible to prevent the dissemination. Other professional opponents of Hahnemann went even further in trying to silence him by approaching the Duke of Köthen. They accused Hahnemann of trying to get his worthless preventive measures against cholera accepted by unsuspecting doctors, and they therefore requested that the Duke have his writings suppressed.

If anyone can be given the credit for being the father of modern immunology it is Dr Samuel Hahnemann, for he believed and proved to the satisfaction of many that if people were to take small doses of camphor they would remain immune from cholera. Nor was this concept pure speculation. Back in 1799 scarlet fever was rampaging through Leipsic, and three members of a family he was treating became stricken, but a girl who usually caught every infection in the neighbourhood somehow remained immune. Hahnemann pondered on this until he realized that she had been receiving small doses of belladonna (deadly nightsade) for another complaint. This triggered off his memory of people who had accidentally eaten belladonna, and how they had shown the same symptoms as others who had contracted scarlet fever. He immediately gave small doses of the plant to other children living in the same house, and the outcome was they did not catch the disease even though they were in regular close contact with others who had it.

From then onwards he used belladonna as a preventive medicine against scarlet fever extensively, and was repeatedly attacked by other physicians for doing so. Nevertheless time was on his side, and in 1838, the government of Saxony recognized that belladonna had both a preventive and curative role to play in countering scarlet fever, and it ordered that small homeopathic doses should be administered whenever there was an outbreak of the illness.

However, to return to the cholera epidemic of the 1830s, despite the measures taken against his proposed treatment for cholera the news of Hahnemann's work spread, and before long reports began to reach him from far and wide informing him how successful camphor had been. Yet it was from England and

Austria that the documented proof of its value in combating cholera came.

Austria had previously banned the practice of homeopathy by an Imperial Edict instigated by members of the medical profession, but when cholera swept into Vienna in 1836, a priest, Father Veith, who was also a physician, obtained permission for one hospital to try out the homeopathic remedy. The result was that only a third of the patients died in the hospital where homeopathy was used, while two-thirds of the patients died in the other hospitals where the doctors dismissed it as humbug.

England was more fortunate as a Dr F. F. Quinn had travelled through Europe during the cholera epidemics to study both the disease and Hahnemann's methods. When he returned to London he practised homeopathy, and together with some friends established the London Homeopathic Hospital in 1844. Therefore when cholera struck London in 1854 the hospital had the necessary knowledge as to what could be done, leaving the other allopathic doctors at a definite disadvantage because they had no therapeutic means at their disposal, a fact which became evident when the official figures for the epidemic were finally released. The word *finally* is necessary here owing to the machinations of Dr Paris, President of the College of Physicians, a bitter opponent of homeopathy, who used all the means at his disposal to have the true figures of the epidemic suppressed. Finally the efforts of Dr Paris were defeated by Dr Quinn and a group of influential friends, and what emerged was that 54,000 people had died of cholera. Of these, 59.2 per cent had died while receiving the regular, orthodox treatment; while of those treated homeopathically only in 16.4 per cent of cases had the illness proved to be fatal. This led Dr McCloughlin, the Medical Inspector, to say, ' If it should please the Lord to visit me with cholera I would wish to fall into the hands of a homeopathic physician.'[4]

When the Member of Parliament who was responsible for originally suppressing the figures showing the effectiveness of homeopathy in fighting cholera, was asked to give an explanation he lamely commented that he had made the exclusion because if he had done otherwise it might have encouraged quackery!

To people uncontaminated with prejudices the cholera figures would be sufficient to warrant an in-depth investigation into the homeopathic system of medicine. It never happened, as Dr Charles Wheeler made plain when speaking to the British Medical Association: 'To say that the vast body of medical opinion for a hundred years has rejected homeopathy is true, but to imply that it has rejected it after trial and investigation is a gross fallacy. Each successive decade has handed down its prejudice and ignorance on to the next, and the simple tests which would have settled the matter once and for all time have never been made, save by the few, who in consequence have maintained the heresy.'

Neither has there been any investigation in the United States, where homeopathy was introduced by Dr Constantine Hering in the early part of the nineteenth century, although following the First World War, when influenza was sweeping through the United States, the homeopathic practitioners claimed that the mortality rate in the 17,000 patients they had treated was 0.3 per cent, against an orthodox mortality rate among patients of approximately 20 per cent.

Instead of having an open, scientific approach to homeopathy after the cholera figures were released, the British medical profession became even more determined to keep homeopathic doctors from becoming registered under the Medical Registration Bill, even though all of them were qualified physicians.

In the beginning the orthodox scheme to keep the homeopaths from being listed on the Medical Register succeeded in the House of Commons, but failed in the House of Lords, where an amendment was made after a medical student at Aberdeen University was asked if he would give up his interest in homeopathic medicine when he received his degree. The student refused to bow down to the orthodox blackmail, and it was his refusal that led to homeopathic practitioners being rightfully included as Registered Medical Practitioners.

But so much for the history of homeopathy, for it is more important to see how it is alleged to work, and ascertain what its position is in the medical world today.

Perhaps the best way to commence an assessment of it as a form of treatment is to take part of Hahnemann's philosophy that,

'There are no diseases, only patients'; or to quote from an article written by Maggie Brittain: 'How do you like being treated when you're ill – as a mere collection of symptoms . . . or as a complete human being?'[5] For both of these imply that no two people will ever react in exactly the same way to the same illness.

Writing in the British medical magazine *General Practitioner*,[6] Dr D. M. Foubister, BS, MB, ChB, DCH, illustrated how people are more important than a diagnostic label. He quoted two possible reactions to measles in children. One child would perhaps be irritable, suffer from an intense thirst, get annoyed about being fussed over and moved; while another child would demand constant attention, cry a lot, and wanted little to drink. Instead of treating both alike for measles, the first child would receive minute doses of *bryonia* (wild hops), which would normally bring about pains at being moved, irritability, excessive thirst, etc., while the second would receive *pulsatilla* (wind flower), which evokes crying, a fear of being alone, etc.

Whereas rheumatism is a common diagnosis applicable to millions of people the individual reaction to it can be very different, and in homeopathy it is the individual difference, the uniqueness of the individual, that is treated.

To find out what the differences are the homeopath at the initial consultation makes a record of everything about his or her patient – physical characteristics, psychological make-up, job reactions, life-style, and how the illness affects the patient. Given that data the practitioner prescribes a remedy, and often it is found that patients suffering from a host of different diagnostic labels will be given the same medication, as it matches their reactions and not the illness.

Dr Foubister in his article mentions how his non-homeopathic colleagues tend to scoff at homeopathic remedies because the amount of the drug, herb or mineral is too small to be effective when considered alongside the amount they would prescribe, and accordingly any results which are obtained must come from 'the unaided work of nature or faith. If the condition of the patient was serious or recovery virtually impossible, then he – the non-homeopathic physician – argues that a wrong diagnosis must have been made . . .'

The charge of 'faith-healing' isn't new to the homeopath as it was levelled against homeopathy early in the nineteenth century, but it was refuted by Carl von Boenninghausen, a layman who became a disciple of Hahnemann and was such a successful homeopath that in 1843 he was granted permission to practise homeopathic medicine by King Friedrich Wilhelm XIV.

Von Boenninghausen started his career by trying out the remedies on animals, and before long he had a large veterinary practice, and, to quote from his own records, among the cures he obtained was a horse that had been *winded* for nine months, and a 'cow . . . seized with the malignant mouth and hoof disease' – the disastrous foot and mouth. He gave the cow homeopathic doses of arsenic and thuja, and 'In eight days she was perfectly restored.'

When I set out to write this book I too thought homeopathy was akin to faith-healing, and therefore it was quite a shock when I interviewed a Mr Stan Duncombe, a manipulative therapist in Coventry. He told me how he had been forced to make a study of homeopathy as he felt that, while manipulative therapy was efficient, unless his patients were physically and psychologically ready to make a recovery, 'I could make the physical adjustments, but if the body is not at the stage when it is healthy, he or she would have to keep on coming back for further adjustments,' and the homeopathic dosage fulfilled his requirements.

My interview with Stan Duncombe was interesting, and I was about to switch off the tape recorder when he casually mentioned that he had recently extended his manipulative therapy practice to animals.

A veterinary surgeon had asked him if he would consider manipulating the spines of five racing greyhounds who were in need since the speed at which they ran around the race-track placed tremendous pressure on the spine and led to spinal displacements. More as an experiment than anything else Mr Duncombe agreed to examine the dogs and they were duly brought to his clinic. Each dog was muzzled in turn before it was lifted onto the treatment couch, and the spinal displacements were located and adjusted. The result of the manipulation was that when they next raced all of them had increased speed and won their race. As that was sufficient proof for the veterinarian the dogs were brought back for further treatment, only on their second and subsequent visits they did not need muzzling. 'It was just as if they knew what I was doing to them was making them feel better, and they stood quite still while I manipulated their spines,' Mr Duncombe said.

As he was on the point of leaving, the veterinarian asked, jokingly, if Stan Duncombe could help him with another greyhound in his charge who suffered from an 'anxiety neurosis'; whenever the dog was put with other greyhounds it showed signs of fear, and tried to get as far away from them as it could. This anxiety meant that whenever the dog was raced it would run wide to avoid close contact with the other dogs racing, and consequently never won any of the races it was entered for. Again on an experimental basis Mr Duncombe gave the vet a homeopathic preparation discovered by Dr Edward Bach, called the 'rescue' remedy, together with instructions to put it into the dog's drinking water three times a day.[7] The vet found that Duncombe had worked a miracle once more, and the dog, who had no way of knowing what orthodox medicine thought of the Bach remedies, lost its anxiety syndrome, and in its next race ran among the other dogs, emerging as the winner at the finishing line.

I told the manipulative therapist that I thought the case of the formerly anxiety-prone dog was far more convincing as proof of the efficacy of homeopathy than all the human case histories he had mentioned, because the dog was unaware it was receiving treatment in its drinking water. He looked at me a little askance until it dawned upon him what I was getting at: that it ruled out any possibility of the cure being the result of verbal suggestion or faith-healing in the usually accepted sense of the term.

Some time after my trip to Coventry I happened to mention the case of the greyhound to a well-known homeopath, and she was not in the least surprised. She told me about two budgerigars, one of which became morose and dejected after its companion died. The homeopath decided what she would give to a human being stricken with remorse, and added a few drops of the selected remedy to the bird's drinking-water. Within half an hour the budgerigar had recovered its former well-being and was singing away happily.

As this animal evidence tends to rule out the faith-healing accusation, the next argument mentioned by Dr Foubister was the escape route often used by members of the orthodoxy when homeopathy has worked: 'the condition must have been wrongly diagnosed.' If this excuse is to be accepted, and it is the stock answer when alternative medical practitioners obtain results after allopathic medicine has failed, this must imply that the methods of diagnosis used by the registered practitioners are sadly lacking in accuracy, and that something should be done to rectify them.

Even if the question of wrong diagnosis occurred infrequently in orthodox medicine, the homeopaths state that it shows the weakness of the system, for the registered orthodox physician has to collate all the symptoms, and then find the label of the illness before he can treat it. The homeopath is freed from this pitfall because he or she is not interested in putting labels onto people's symptoms. This difference was well illustrated in the case of a patient who had been in a coma for several days without the specialists being able to diagnose what the exact cause was; hence no treatment could be prescribed. When the hospital staff were at a complete loss a homeopath was called in, and while he had no idea as to what caused the coma, something he wasn't interested in, he assured everyone he would be able to assist the patient. Taking the coma as the main reaction to the illness, and knowing that large doses of opium would put people into a coma, the homeopath prescribed small amounts of opium, and the patient rapidly recovered consciousness.

Still looking at the opposing methods of treatment, the simple tonsilectomy operation, which has been recommended by thousands of doctors and carried out on millions of people for enlarged and enflamed tonsils, may have been unnecessary as the conditions the operation is meant to rectify respond well to homeopathy without surgical intervention. Some followers of Hahnemann have shown that up to 95 per cent of all the cases seen by them have been cured without surgery, a fact confirmed by the late Dr J. P. Compton Burnett, who stated, 'There are a good many homeopathic remedies for enlarged tonsils, and thousands of cases . . . have been cured . . .' But these alleged cures have been summarily dismissed without scientific investigation, and some time ago a doctor had his name erased from the Medical Register for claiming that enlarged tonsils could be treated without surgery.

At a more serious level, a married woman had an enormous tumour on the left ovary which made her stomach look as if she was nine months pregnant. Her general physical condition was poor, and she had a temperature of 104.5 degrees fahrenheit. The orthodox physicians informed her that immediate surgery was necessary if she was to have any chance at all, and even then there was a strong chance she would not survive. But a homeopath, Dr S. E. Chapman was called in and studied the overall symptomatology before prescribing minute dosages. In two days the woman's temperature was down to normal, with most of the acute symptoms resolved. Fourteen days later she was able to sit up in a chair, and after six months she was completely cured, and free from any signs of the former tumour.[8]

Homeopathic literature abounds with thousands upon thousands of documented case histories like the one above I have just quoted. I doubt if all of them can be dismissed with the derisive comment that 'they were incorrectly diagnosed'. But if we leave organic illnesses at this point, and turn to the possible role that homeopathy could play in treating anxiety and depression, the same favourable results come to light.

I talked to Mrs Valerie Gilmore, a manipulative therapist with a practice at Cowley, Oxford, who like Mr Duncombe came to the conclusion that she needed to incorporate homeopathy into her work to obtain the best results for her patients. Living in the old university city it is hardly surprising that she has a large number of students and members of the college faculties coming to see her, with tension, anxiety and depression.

She said that the majority of the students tended to be in their third and final year and ready to take their final examinations, and under those stressful circumstances the regular tranquillizers and anti-depressants had little effect. Yet, when she prescribed homeopathic remedies and relaxed them physically through depth-massage they quickly became stress-free and able to continue studying. Mrs Gilmore also found that the same applied to the many people who visited her because they were unable to sleep.

The remedies given by homeopaths are 'simples' – comprised of a small dose of a single drug, herb, mineral or other substance; they have proved over the last hundred years to be non-toxic and non-habit-forming; they do not give rise to iatrogenic illnesses, and are comparatively inexpensive when compared to the cost of many chemical drug preparations. For these reasons it is time the British National Health Service, which is financed by the public, ordered stringent trials of homeopathic remedies both in the best interests of public health and to save public money.

Yet what is actually happening to the Hahnemann system of medicine today?

There are now fewer registered homeopathic doctors in Britain than there were at the time of the cholera epidemic in the nineteenth century, and although they may not like my assessment of their present situation, the homeopaths have only themselves to blame. Their anxiety to remain within the ranks of orthodox medicine, and not to be associated with heterodox practitioners, has driven them into a position from which they cannot advance.

The orthodox medical profession either dismisses them as cranks or opposes them as a group to be fought. A general practitioner and homeopath, Dr Johana Brieger, tried to explain why this happened to Elizabeth Anstice, Features Editor of *World Medicine*:[9] 'By the time a medical student qualifies he has undertaken six or seven years of brainwashing into the behaviour and attitudes of orthodox medicine. Even if he feels like doing further training he is hardly likely to consider homeopathy; perhaps when he is older and has been in practice long enough to become dissatisfied and disillusioned with orthodox medicine he may start looking round for alternatives and wonder about homeopathy. But there is no financial incentive for him to change.'

Obviously there is a lot of truth in what Dr Brieger said, but she omitted to quote from the anti-homeopathy propaganda which is aimed at doctors. One example was a broadsheet entitled 'Beyond Belief – A Review of the Irrational in Medicine' which was published by Geigy (UK) Limited in 1970, and sent to every General Practitioner in Britain.

Under the title 'The History of Medical Sects' the editors introduced Professor Ackerknecht's contribution as '. . . a review of the more bizarre forms of healing . . .', and that can hardly be considered as a scientific introduction to a system of medicine.

The Professor showed that the various sects, including homeopathy, were a revolt against blood-letting, purging and other ineffective and offensive measures carried out by orthodox physicians of the past, and came into being as more acceptable alternatives. 'As long as he was getting better the patient found the foolish theories of the sectarians acceptable; that they might at times be dangerous only became apparent later.' (Hence Professor Ackerknecht might have added that the latter part of his sentence could equally be applied to modern sectarians of the pill-cult!)

In the section devoted to homeopathy the Professor makes the sweeping and derogatory statement, 'Like many who practise psychosomatic medicine they (the homeopaths) have remained formally within scientific medicine, although they renounce it in principle because homeopathic diagnosis is "intuitive".' A few lines below he quotes Wunderlich, who said of homeopathy in 1859, 'Criticism of Hahnemann's doctrine appears completely superfluous. A plain and unvarnished account of it is enough to condemn it without need for anything more.' However, the Professor admitted that until the middle of the nineteenth century a patient was perhaps better off seeking treatment from a homeopath as he would otherwise have been bled or poisoned to death, but he added, 'Homeopathy lived for a long time on the credit it had then gained as well as on the human preference for the absurd . . .'

Professor Ackerknecht condemned Hahnemann's system of medicine as 'intuitive' and therefore unscientific, yet his own remarks could be considered equally intuitive and unscientific, because he made no reference to any trials made of homeopathic remedies to support his statements, but apparently preferred to rely upon his expert knowledge. It was nearly enough to make me rush round to my GP and get a quickly written out prescription for tranquillizers . . . but not quite!

8

Nature Holds the Cure - Naturopathy

Although there is a definite gulf and considerable antagonism separating the herbalist and the homeopath from their allopathic medical counterparts there is a far wider breach, and a far greater degree of enmity, between the registered medical practitioner and the naturopathic physician. For the Naturopath not only rejects the very basis of modern orthodox medicine, but considers the methodology and pharmacological approach to illness to be harmful to the future health of anyone treated with drugs.

One may try to simplify the medical philosophy that motivates the naturopath: if a patient with a severe cold goes to see his General Practitioner, and complains of all the usual symptoms (a running nose, watering eyes, heavy sweating, excessive mucus in the throat, a feeling of lethargy), the GP is trained to recognize that his patient has been infected by a cold virus and is in need of a prescription for a chemically compounded drug to kill the virus. What is prescribed may be nothing more than codeine – an alkaloid originally obtained from poppy juice – but once the symptoms have disappeared the doctor considers the patient to be cured.

However, if the patient with the same cold chose to visit a naturopath, the naturopathic practitioner would have explained to him that the symptoms were Nature's way of trying to rid the body of impurities previously accumulated in the system, and that the symptoms were therefore beneficial to his future well-being.

The treatment the naturopath would prescribe would be aimed at assisting the body to eliminate the over-load of toxins through a short period of fasting, and perhaps of hot Epsom-salt baths to encourage sweating.

If the eliminative process is hindered, as the naturopath's claim it is by the GP, then the toxins remain within the body building up until the poison level reaches the stage where the functioning of the body is affected, thus causing disease. Hence the accusation that any form of suppressive drug therapy is a hazard to health.

I talked to a leading naturopath about the common cold, and he enlarged upon the medical concept by saying that auto-intoxication of the human organism is the result of many factors. Eating too much of the wrong foods containing chemical preservatives or tainted with chemical insecticides, and eating too much meat and animal fats instead of adhering to a healthy diet were factors. Another was that due to an incorrect diet and lack of exercise many people became constipated, and constipation means that the body does not have the opportunity to regularly discharge waste materials, so the waste builds up inside the organism increasing the internal pollution. Finally he commented upon the effect of stress on the individual, which he and other adherents of Nature Cure maintain also increases the internal poisons and prevents natural anal elimination.

To prove to me that the hypothesis he was presenting was valid he explained why people had more colds in winter than in summer. According to him, during the summer we all sweat a lot owing to the warm temperature, and as we sweat, the toxins, the impurities we have amassed within us in various ways, are continually being eliminated via the millions of pores in the skin. If we get a summer cold the reason he gave was this: should anyone find themselves in a cold draught, or should the body be submitted to damp coldness, this quick change of temperature makes the pores close up to preserve body heat; when the pores close up rapidly the discharge of toxins from within the body is prevented, and as this waste has to come out in one way or another, it uses the unaffected eliminative organs such as the nose, eyes, etc.

It appeared on the surface to be a rational explanation, but his theory had one glaring omission; it failed to take into account the virus infections. I challenged the naturopath on this. Didn't he admit that at times people were infected by alien and virulent microbes, such as the virus which caused the Asian flu epidemics which rampaged across the world not too long ago? He had an answer ready for me which I have since discovered is the foundation upon which Nature Cure practitioners base their entire work.

'To answer your question it is necessary for me to ask you a couple of questions in return. "Where does the virus originally come from, and why is it that certain people have immunity?" He did not give me time to formulate an answer even if I could have done so, which I couldn't. Instead he quoted what one of the discoverers of the germ theory, Professor Virchow had written prior to his death, 'If I could live my life over again I would devote it to proving that germs *seek* their natural *habitat* – diseased tissue – rather than being the *cause* of the diseased tissue, e.g. mosquitoes *seek* the stagnant water, but do not *cause* the pool to become stagnant.'[1]

The naturopath continued, 'From what Virchow wrote you can see that the original virus comes from inside a person who has allowed his or her system to become filled with toxic material, and then the virus goes on to infect only those other people whose systems are also ready to act as breeding grounds; people who are, to use the Virchow quote, 'internally stagnant already.'

And that is the crux of naturopath medicine, that the 'germ theory' originated by Virchow and Pasteur is a fallacy, and that what the two scientists had seen through their microscopes – the microbes present in a diseased body – were erroneously accepted by both of them to mean that the microbes were the cause of the disease rather than being the result of it.

The type of error which the naturopath claim Virchow and Pasteur made is not new. Not too long ago the medical profession believed that masturbation, 'self-abuse', could be a cause of insanity, and the conclusion (later proved to be incorrect as masturbation does nothing more than give the masturbator a stronger right or left arm depending upon whether he or she is right- or left-handed) was arrived at through observing mental patients in the earlier mental hospitals – lunatic asylums – openly masturbating. Then the observers put the cart before the horse. Instead of realizing that it was the mental problems afflicting the patients that made them try to ease the internal tensions through masturbation, they assumed masturbation was the causative agent.

In addition to claiming that Virchow earlier in his career reached the wrong conclusions, the naturopaths claim that Louis Pasteur, in addition to being wrong in his findings, had unscrupulously plagiarized the work of Professor Antoine Béchamp (1816–1908) on microbiology, and had also misunderstood the principles he pirated. As this is a serious accusation, and if it were found to be correct then allopathic medicine would be marching along the wrong road, I decided to have a look at the work of Professor Béchamp as outlined in his book *The Blood and its Third Anatomical Element*.[2]

The introduction to Béchamp's book was written by a Dr Montague R. Leverson, MD, PhD, MA, and Leverson confirmed the naturopaths' assertions. He showed how and when Pasteur did his plagiarism, and quoted Professor Béchamp as saying that he – Béchamp – hoped that the 'Microbian Theory of Disease' would soon be relegated to the garbage can as it was the 'greatest scientific silliness of the age'.

All this is indeed alarming, and it becomes even more frightening when confronted with other indisputable facts with which the Nature Cure practitioners are anxious to confront the interested enquirer.

Biologists everywhere admit that inside every human body there are millions of microbes or germs which are essential to the maintenance of good health. Some of these are lethal when taken from their natural environment, such as the bugs that have their habitat in the intestines. Of course these rarely cause any trouble, but at times they can and do get out of control and commence attacking the lining of the intestines, and when that occurs the body becomes ill.

As the internal microbes have an obvious part to play in

breaking down dead and dying tissue and toxic materials, if this knowledge is carried to its logical conclusion it appears, at least to me, to be an inescapable fact that all of us carry within ourselves the seeds of our own destruction – our own future illnesses – and we can quite possibly make ourselves ill any time we wish to by abusing the laws of nature. This idea that people can make themselves ill is unpalatable to many, so it should not come as a surprise that it was Béchamp's ideas which were relegated to the garbage can, and Pasteur's which were found to be more acceptable. By accepting the Pasteur principle man can escape from being held responsible for his own diseased state and claim, whenever he is smitten by an illness, 'I have been attacked and invaded by foreign germs. Doctor, please kill the horrible little things for me so that I can be well again.'

Long before I decided to write this book on Alternative Medicine and the theoretical considerations behind the various drugless therapies, I talked to a famous psychiatrist from New York City, Dr Gotthard Booth, MD, while he was on a visit to Britain. We were discussing the possible causes of cancer as we were driving along looking at the countryside, and he told me that he was sure, and his research had given confirmation, that cancer was psychosomatic and was created within the human organism by stress, when the individual felt he could not continue living within the restricted life-style encompassing him at the time. Dr Booth went on to say that if the cancer patient's psychological attitude towards life could be changed he was equally sure the natural resistance of the body could become re-activated and the cancer could remit. He gave me details of case histories to substantiate the point he was making. Then he made what I feel to be a very profound statement, and I only wish I had had a tape recorder running as he spoke, but I didn't and shall have to rely upon my memory: 'Peter, this is where current cancer research is wrong. They are continuing to look for the virus which causes cancer instead of seeing that the seeds of cancer are inside all of us and can be activated at any time. And more important still this is why people want a cancer virus to be found, because then they won't have to face up to the fact that they inflict cancer upon themselves . . .'

Miss June Johns, a well-known author and friend of mine, made some pertinent comments on the same theme when we were discussing the origins of illness.

She had found while doing research for her animal books, *The Mating Game*,[3] and *Zoo Without Bars*,[4] that certain animals have inside them parasites and viruses that remain in balance until the animals are put under stress. Then, when the animal is confronted with a stressful situation, the parasites begin to take over, and unless something is done to help the animal, it quickly dies.

Miss Johns wrote about wallabies and kangaroos:

> In zoos they breed readily but show signs of temperament that can have alarming results. Most animals, including man, harbour germs and viruses which do no harm unless conditions of stress cause them to multiply. Kangeroos and wallabies are susceptible to Lumpy Jaw, and unless it is diagnosed very quickly and treated with antibiotics, it gets such a hold that it is almost fatal or the animal has to be put down to prevent its suffering. Sometimes the cause of the stress is obvious, as with hundreds of joeys that are brought annually to Australian zoos by people who have shot the mothers and taken pity on the helpless young. But even those born in zoos allow themselves to succumb to Lumpy Jaw if they are disturbed. It might be their removal to a different paddock, or even disruption of the routine each autumn when the herd is sexed. Keepers have to handle them gently and quietly, or within days half the animals will fall victim to Lumpy Jaw.
>
> Occasionally there is no apparent cause, but an examination usually reveals that the flesh of the jaws is riddled with a fungus-like infection.[5]

The same applies to camels and more particularly to penguins, and June Johns told me the history of the lung disease that kills many of them once they have been handled by humans.

As long as they were on land penguins had no fear of man in the beginning. Their only enemies were in the sea, and until fifty years ago when explorers and sailors discovered their existence they would waddle right up to a man and allow themselves to be handled and touched. But after humans began killing them and capturing them to be taken to zoos as exhibits the penguins learned, within a few generations, that man was the creature to be feared most of all and avoided whenever possible.

Being frightened of man, penguins have to be chased and caught, and until a few years ago the most common way of catching them was to run and throw a sack over the selected victim. As they are birds, the sudden darkness of the sack caused stress, and it was found when the birds arrived at their destination that they were either dead or suffering from a disease where the lungs were infected with a type of fungus which prevented them from breathing and brought about death due to suffocation. It was first thought that the sacking must contain an allergic substance which caused the parasitic fungus, so different methods of catching penguins were tried. But it did not matter what method was employed: when the birds were frightened the parasites inside them became activated and the illness appeared.

Similarly, Dr Janet Harker of Girton College, Cambridge, found that when she caused stress in cockroaches by disturbing their innate sense of time and activity, they developed malignant, cancerous tumours.

Yet, to return to the human animal and his illnesses, while the naturopaths accept that stress can play a part in engendering disease, they consider the major source to be the internal pollution due to incorrect diet.

To non-Nature Cure people the idea that diet can cause disease has been a source of ridicule. Vegetarians have been a constant source of many comedians jokes, and the 'nut-eaters' were considered to be 'nuts' who needed putting away. Now the amusement is beginning to abate, at least in certain allopathic medical circles.

In the monthly *World Medicine*'s Review of the Year, published in 1971, there appeared an article entitled 'Diet and Disease'[6] by the famous surgeon, Mr Denis Burkitt, whom the editors introduced to the readers as a man who 'believes that one of the most important clues to health in the future may lie in a detailed study of diets in underdeveloped countries. He suggests that the association of many of the so-called "diseases of civilization" with simple dietary factors may soon be as clearly defined as the association between smoking and lung cancer.' In his article Mr Burkitt enumerated some of the diseases which may have a correlation between diet and illness, and these included, appendicitis, diverticula, adenomatous polyps, cancer of the colon, obesity, dental caries, diabetes and arthrosclerosis.

Among his conclusions Mr Burkitt wrote to the effect that constipation, prevalent in Britain, is due to a cellulose-depleted diet, and he decried the confusion surrounding the white versus wholemeal flour controversy, which had arisen from 'the multitude of unsubstantiated claims made by many "natural food" exponents and exploited by the health-food shops.' He immediately continued, 'The accumulated incidental accretions which surround and even supersede what is fundamentally important in relation to diet has, in the mind of many, associated the cry for wholemeal flour with a type of paramedical quackery that would consider everything that is processed or "unnatural" as essentially bad.'

More recently at a meeting of the British Medical Association held in Coventry on 28 April 1973, Dr Barry Lewis, a cardiac specialist at the Hammersmith Hospital in London, told the doctors attending that an international survey had shown that Londoners were on the way to eating themselves to death through consuming too much butter, milk, fatty meat and fried foods, and their eating habits led to them having higher cholesterol levels than people living in Naples, Geneva and Uppsala, Sweden.

Looking at the difference of cholesterol levels between Londoners and Neapolitans, who drink more wine and have a lower cholesterol level, Dr Lewis made the comment that it would seem 'booze is less bad than butter'.

The heart specialist also said, 'I don't think it is stress so much as diet that is responsible for the epidemic of heart disease now hitting us,' and his advice to anyone worried about their heart was to use margarine instead of butter, cut down on other dairy products, and, when cooking, use vegetable oils to fry the food in.

Although many would argue with him for dismissing stress as

a major contributing factor in heart disease, Dr Lewis' statement brought an immediate public reaction from the British Milk Marketing Board, which annually spends large sums of money to promote the sale of milk.

'Before mounting our campaigns to promote milk and butter we take expert medical advice,' the Milk Marketing Board countered.

'There is no conclusive proof that animal fats have any connection with heart disease.

'There is no doubt in most people's minds that milk is good for you.'[7]

Obviously the Milk Marketing Board did not listen to all Dr Lewis had to say, because he said that in those patients attending the Hammersmith Hospital's Lipids (Blood Fats) Clinic who had followed his advice, the cholesterol level fell by a quarter, and the levels of other blood fats were halved.

While allopathic medicine may be split over the diet-equals-illness debate, the naturopaths have no doubts in their minds about the effects of popular eating habits, hence the first part of any naturopathic treatment is nearly always a period of fasting; doing without food to let the body cleanse itself.

The naturopath has been taught that *all* illnesses stem from internal pollution or toxification; so the name given to a set of symptoms by the registered practitioner does not have the same significance for him, and he does not think or say he has the ability or knowledge to cure anything. Instead he accepts that nature will accomplish it if the patient will allow the body to function naturally.

Why is the fast so important to them?

There is a two-part answer to this question.

Nature Cure followers say it is natural. Animals and babies do not eat when they are ill, and if it assists their return to health then it must assist human adults.

The second part of their answer is that by stopping the intake of food the body is freed to deal with the accumulated toxic materials which have been piling up inside it through misguided eating habits, through stress or perhaps injury to the physical structure of the body.

H

To assist nature eliminate the toxins, the breeding grounds for the virus, enemas and colonic irrigation may be used, together with a selected type of water-treatment – hydrotherapy.

At the Tyringham Naturopath Clinic I saw how water can be used therapeutically. A patient was wrapped in a white sheet that had previously been soaked in cold water, and then he was enclosed in blankets. Hot-water bottles were put around the patient, and he was left in his wrap for a long time. When the treatment was completed the formerly white sheet was heavily stained with extensive, foul-smelling brown marks, and the Medical Director of the Clinic, Mr Sidney Rose-Neil, assured me the stains were indelible and the sheet would have to be destroyed. Having seen all the brown, stinking material coming from the pores of what had previously seemed to be a clean body, it struck me that it was not beyond the realms of possibility that all of us in the future will have this type of internal cleansing occasionally as a part of preventive medicine.

Physical manipulation may also form a part of the naturopathic treatment if deemed necessary, but a new and carefully chosen diet to match the patient's condition is always recommended.

It all sounds too simple for words. Yet does it work?

The naturopaths assert that it does. Once the detoxification regime has been completed, and any necessary manipulation has been done, the viruses, germs, microbes and harmful bacteria will, according to them, disappear. They will present case histories as evidence, and some of them are remarkable. There was a published case of a 23-year-old girl who went to see a naturopath and medical herbalist, Mr Eric F. Powell, ND, with tuberculosis of the lungs in such an advanced state that she had been informed by orthodox specialists that she would be dead within a year, or shortly afterwards.

Mr Powell informed the girl's mother that he could offer little hope as she was in an advanced stage with frequent haemorrhages. The mother implored him to try as he was their last hope.

Putting the girl on to a diet, together with specific herbal remedies, Mr Powell used the *Baunscheidt Method* of piercing the skin of the abdomen and spine with multiple needles and then rubbing into the pierced areas the specified oil. Pus, the toxic waste, started pouring out of the body.

Every third week Mr Powell sent a sputum specimen to the Ministry of Health for analysis, and the first three reports came back stating the sputum showed heavy concentrations of bacteria. The fourth report, however, came back as negative, and subsequent reports said there was no sign of the tubercle bacilli.

As the young female had been treated by Mr Powell thirty years before he wrote up her case in *Fitness and Health Through Herbs*,[8] and he kept in contact with her family for many years afterwards, thereby ensuring the tuberculosis was not reactivated at a later date, this cure is impressive.

Since I have mentioned the Baunscheidt Method above, it is possible the reader wonders what it is. I did myself when I read Mr Powell's case initially. It was discovered in 1848 by the German, Carl Baunscheidt, while he was suffering from gout in the right hand and arm which caused him intense pain and prevented him from working.

He was sitting in the garden one day when an insect stung him on his gouty hand. The hand became red and the skin began to discharge a fluid, but later Baunscheidt found his gout had gone. He developed this concept under the name of 'Dermato-biotikon', taken from the Greek and meaning 'skin-reviver', and came to the conclusion that unless the impurities within the body were expelled through the skin healing could not take place.

In the book *Der Baunscheidtismus*[9] a German doctor, George Alfred Tienes, who became a naturopathic physician explained how the treatment worked, and gave many case histories in support of the theory. One of these related to Dr Ino Meier of McKeesport, Pa., USA, who developed tuberculosis of the spine when he was thirty years old. None of Meier's medical colleagues could offer him any hope of recovery, and it was a priest who suggested that he try the 'skin-reviver' method. There resulted the exudation of pus through the skin, and after four months of the treatment Dr Meier was well enough to return to medical practice and to become the leading advocate of the therapy in the United States.

Later Dr Meier said, 'In my twenty-four years of practice, I have used Baunscheidtismus in numberless cases, especially in rheumatism and paralyses, gout, lumbago, eye inflammation, gangrene, skin diseases and syphilis, scrofulous conditions, neuralgias, etc., and have had splendid successes. Even in the most stubborn cases the results have been wonderful.'

Of course the orthodox medical profession can dismiss these examples in the same way that they ridicule the anti-virus theory, but in the United States the reaction of the American Medical Association has often been more drastic. By looking at what happened to Dr Alice Chase, DC, who died at her home in Nyack, New York, in April 1973, the AMA antagonism becomes apparent.

Dr Chase was active in emphasizing the importance of diet and was the author of the book *Nutrition for Health*. She obtained a doctorate in osteopathy from an American osteopathic medical school, and in keeping with naturopathic ideas advocated that people who were sick should be assisted by natural means to eliminate the causative poisons from their systems, while publicly maintaining that the use of drugs was harmful.

Her professional views on illness annoyed the allopathic organization, and to quote from a report on her death appearing in *The Daily Telegraph*,[10] 'The American Medical Association retaliated by questioning her methods. She was forced to close her nursing home and, two years ago, *Nutrition for Health* was banned.'

The newspaper item was possibly the understatement of the year, for when its New York correspondent, Mabel Elliott, wrote, 'The American Medical Association retaliated by *questioning* her methods' from what she wrote afterwards the 'questioning' amounted to her clinic being forcibly closed, and her book being banned to prevent anyone from making up their own minds about the value or stupidity of the contents.

From this it would appear that in the 'Land of the Free', where competition is considered to be healthy (no pun intended) and an essential part of the country's basic liberty, this does not apply to medicine, and that certain unelected people have the power to decide, in the best dictatorial fashion, what information is best for the masses!

If a note of bitterness is detected in the previous paragraph it is because, as the reader will already be aware, I too ran into medical censorship in the United States while trying to gather material for this book. Hoxsey could not send me details of his book, nor could Dr William Donald Kelley, DDS.

Just why I was surprised now puzzles me. Had I thought about it all more carefully I would have recalled how, back in the 1950s, the books of Dr Wilhelm Reich, MD, were burned because they contained data about his experimental work with cancer and his using what he called an Orgone Accumulator as a therapeutic aid. As I have never used a Reich accumulator I am unable to give any opinion, but I did resent being unable to buy a copy of Reich's book, *Cancer Biopathy*, because someone had decided for me that I should not read it.

Yet, as this chapter comes to a close it would be remiss of me leave the impression that the conflict is limited to a battle between allopathic and naturopathic medicine. For there is another struggle going on simultaneously, between the *orthodox* naturopaths who consider the use of herbal medicine and homeopathy to border upon heresy. This faction's view was expressed by Mr Harry Benjamin, a member of the British Naturopathic Association and author of many books on natural healing, when he wrote, 'It is true that herbalism is, in many ways, to be preferred to orthodox medicine, but that does not allow it to rank with Nature Cure treatment. The genuine Naturopath does *not* make use of herbalism in his work . . .' A little later he mentioned the use of the Schuessler Biochemic treatment, which gives the patient what Dr Schuessler considered to be the essential tissue salts in homeopathic dosages: 'As a general rule, however, the use of even these slight additional aids to healing is not desirable. The patient must be made to understand that it is the *natural forces within himself which do the work of healing,* not external aids and appurtenances which come out of a bottle or capsule.'[11]

The views of the *unorthodox* naturopaths was best summed up by Mr Eric F. Powell, ND, who is also an authority on herbal medicine, when he was asked why he used various therapies when working with a patient. 'Many are the conditions where herbs alone can cure, but in a number progress can be speeded up by the employment of other sane and harmless methods in addition . . . Of course it is right that we use all methods of healing that are in harmony with natural law and that produce results . . .'[12]

Whether, in the final analysis, naturopathic medicine is a viable and reliable alternative must depend upon a personal decision. For my own part I took a group of mature students studying applied psychology to the Tyringham Naturopathic Clinic some time ago to get their collective opinion. The medical director arranged for them to have lectures on naturopathy and osteopathy, and to mingle with the patients in residence so they could discuss with them their ailments and the treatment being given – treatments that ranged through the entire gamut of drugless medicine: chiropractic, massage, hydrotherapy, osteopathy, physiotherapy . . . The students were then permitted and encouraged by the director to experience certain of the treatments to see if they found them to be beneficial.

At the end of our one and a half day visit to the clinic we all met as a group to try and reach a decision.

As the group's main interest was in applied psychology it was not altogether surprising that its initial conclusion was that, since the naturopaths recognize that stress can play an important part in any illness, the group felt it was a serious omission in the treatment that psychotherapy or medical counselling was not used by the naturopath.

In trying to assess the therapeutic value, the group was equally divided. Half its members said that the patients they had talked to told them that they had derived more benefit from naturopathy than from the treatment received from their own registered doctors. This section of the group also stated that they felt they had personally benefited from the various treatments they had tried, and therefore they were bound to conclude that naturopathy was a valid form of medical therapy. The other half had very strong doubts about everything they had seen and heard. To them, many of the patients were suffering from psychosomatic conditions which would respond to any form of therapy.

When this opinion was voiced the students in opposition challenged them: 'If that assumption is correct, why didn't the patients respond to orthodox medical treatment?' And it was at this point that the group found unanimity. It unanimously agreed that the naturopathic practitioners they had met showed the patients that they cared about them, and as most of the patients interviewed were suffering from chronic diseases and had been told by their own allopathic doctors that nothing more could be done to help them, the naturopaths had told them that this wasn't true. They offered the patients hope by using forms of therapy which had been used successfully with others having the same illnesses and as Dr Axel Munthe said, 'There is no drug as powerful as hope.'

Perhaps an American doctor, Joseph K. Kaplowe, MD, should have the last word: 'When the laboratory can produce the petals of a rose, science will deserve the right to assume the superior attitude prevailing today.' Until then 'Scientific research must be subservient to Natural Law.'

9

Begin at the Back - Osteopathy

In the entire spectrum of heterodox therapies, osteopathy has the distinction of having survived numerous attacks upon it by the allopathic medical profession, and instead of being vanquished has emerged to be accepted by the public as an integral part of the current medical scene.

In Britain more and more people are ceasing to visit their General Practitioner whenever they have any problems with their backs; instead they consult their nearest osteopath, whom they have accepted as being a specialist in spinal and skeletal disorders. This level of acceptance has now reached the stage where many registered doctors are advising certain of their patients to go and see an osteopath, although this recommending of a patient to see an unregistered practitioner is strictly forbidden by the General Medical Council and could result, if the rule were enforced, in the errant allopathic doctor being struck off the Medical Register and prevented from practising in the future.

This tacit recognition by individual doctors does not mean that the majority are prepared to accept osteopaths. Far from it. A large proportion of the orthodox medical fraternity still consider them to be quacks. However, the conservative opposition may be caused by more than a mere hint of jealousy, because the osteopath frequently treats cases which have previously been assessed as incurable, and when he gets results in those instances the blow to the registered doctor's pride is not easily shrugged aside.

Just how this can happen becomes clear when looking at the case of the young Royal Air Force pilot whose spine was badly injured after his aircraft crashed. He was kept in hospital for a long time, and given all the orthodox treatments which should, by medical tenets, have brought about a cure. Nevertheless, at the end of the hospitalization period the pilot was unable to walk without pain or to bend down quickly and easily. He was given a thorough examination, and informed he would have to be invalided out of the Service. As he still wanted to fly, the man went, more in desperation than anything else, to see an osteopath who, after three treatments, corrected the spinal defects and eliminated the previous difficulties the pilot had had with movement. One would have thought the RAF would have been pleased at his recovery, but the young man had a lot of difficulty in convincing the medical officers that he was fit to return to duty.

The same type of success story can be found in every osteopath's files. In fact I asked one prominent unregistered osteopath – and this distinction is necessary as there are a small number of registered doctors in Britain who have completed a course in osteopathy and practise osteopathic manipulation – if he could give me a number of case histories to support the claim I had repeatedly heard: namely that, where skeletal and muscular illnesses were concerned, the registered practitioner and orthopaedic specialists were innocent babes in the wood, doing more harm than good, whereas the osteopath could cure patients in a comparatively short period of time. He was pleased to open his files to me so that I could select anything I wanted, but his immediate response was: 'Personally, I would find it impossible to do what you intend trying, because nearly all the patients coming to see me have been allopathic rejects, and if you want to you can quote me on that.'

I understand what he meant from a personal experience when I was eleven years old. I was flat-footed, and used to walk like Charles Chaplin, with my feet splayed out like the hands of a clock at a quarter to three. The prognosis of our General Practitioner was poor. He informed my mother I would always be the same as I had curvature of the spine. When I heard what he had to say it was a bitter blow because it was my ambition at the time to enter the Royal Navy, and my flat feet would automatically disqualify my entry on medical grounds. Maybe I was just an obstinate child, but I kept on pestering my mother to find someone who could do something to help me. Eventually I was taken to see a lady osteopath in North London and she was sure my spine and feet could be corrected by manipulation and exercises. She was as good as her word. When the time came for me to enter the Navy I was passed medically A1 with no trace of the former flat feet, and to this day I have had no further trouble.

Yet osteopathy has had to pay a large price for its partial acceptance. Its practitioners have had to forget the teachings of the founder of osteopathy, Dr Andrew Taylor Still, which went far beyond the idea of the osteopath being a highly trained extension of the former local 'bone-setter'. Or as one disgruntled osteopath said, 'Most of us have been bribed into accepting a role we were never intended to play.'

To understand what he was trying to explain it is necessary to go back to the beginning of osteopathy, to Dr Still's rejection of the drug-oriented medicine of his period, following the death of three of his children from spinal meningitis.

His search for an alternative medical system led him to accept that people became ill, or prone to illness, if they were structurally unsound, primarily if there was a displacement of the spine. The theory he evolved was that if there was any spinal defect – the osteopathic lesion or subluxation – this would prevent the free flow of blood through the body, and to specific organs. If the life-force inside people, the blood, was impeded, he postulated this would cause an alteration of functioning elsewhere, which in turn would cause disease or allow the body to become diseased.

In his autobiography Dr Still wrote:

In the year 1874 I proclaimed that a disturbed artery marked the beginning to the hour and a minute when disease began to sow its seeds of destruction in the human body; that in no case could it be done [could the disease occur] without a broken or suspended current of arterial blood, which by Nature was intended to supply and nourish all nerves, ligaments, muscles, skin, bones and the artery itself . . .

He was more explicit when he stated:

The rule of the artery must be absolute, universal, unob-
structed, or disease will result. I proclaimed then and there
that all nerves depend wholly on the arterial system for their
qualities such as sensation, nutrition and motion, even though
by the law of reciprocity they furnish force, nutrition and
motion to the artery itself.

When Still accepted that illness was the result of the frame-
work of the physical body being damaged in some way, it became
crystal clear to him that if he could detect and correct the fault
the natural recuperative power of the organism would be freed
to bring about remission. Henceforth, when people came to him
with the full range of normal medical complaints he would commence his examination at the back, at the spinal column, find the
displacement and manipulate it back into its rightful position.

He developed techniques to make the manipulation easier; he
saw the final results in his patients; and, armed with the knowledge he had gleaned together with his theory, Dr Andrew T.
Still established the now renowned College of Osteopathy in
Kirksville, Missouri, in 1892.

And it is the all-embracing osteopathic theory that the allopaths
want the osteopaths to forget. They do not object too loudly or
strongly if the osteopath continues to manipulate the spine and
other parts of the body, assisting sufferers of the 'slipped disc
syndrome', which they have made popular but rarely can do
anything to correct. Yet let an osteopath say, as some of them
do who still adhere to the original Still teachings, that they can
be of assistance in cases of diabetes, asthma, migraine, sinusitis,
constipation, nervous disorders, infertility in both men and
women, or a host of other medical conditions, then they try to
put their orthodox feet down hard.

The price of acceptance and prosperity which the American
osteopaths had to pay was to be taken over, and incorporated
into the ranks of the orthodoxy. This was possibly due to their
training being on a par with that undertaken by allopathic

students, with osteopathic theory and application forming a type of specialism.

Instead of remaining content to be heterodox practitioners, the US osteopaths became more and more orthodox in the course of their struggle for endorsement, so that now, in many of the States of America, there are no longer any Doctors of Osteopathy, those who were formerly in osteopathic practice having exchanged their DO diplomas for that of a Doctor of Medicine, an MD.

Here in the United Kingdom the situation is less straightforward. There is the London School of Osteopathy, whose students ultimately become members of the British Osteopathic Association, but these are post-graduates who are drawn from the Medical Register and who wish to add osteopathic manipulation to their orthodox medical armamentarium.[1] Then there are various organizations training the unregistered practitioner, like the British School of Osteopathy, the British College of Naturopathy and Osteopathy, and a few others.

Having outlined the training organizations available it becomes more complex to unravel the work of the heterodox osteopaths. Some of them restrict their work to what is generally considered to be osteopathy: the correction of skeletal and muscular conditions which result from trauma, etc. Others include naturopathy and treat the complete range of clinical illnesses but frown upon the use of any medicament. There are those who continue to accept Dr Still's teachings that all diseases respond to manipulation; and then there are others who can only be described as 'eclectic osteopathic practitioners', who use homeopathic, herbal and similar alternative therapeutic systems such as acupuncture whenever they feel it would be beneficial to their patients.

Finally there is a new type of heterodox therapist appearing in the British medical field: those who refer to themselves as manipulative therapists, and as far as I have been able to ascertain the majority of these have received their training at the Northern Institute of Massage, in Blackpool, Lancashire.

As the name of their *alma mater* suggests, these therapists commenced learning massage and basic manipulative techniques to assist them in their chosen career as physical therapists. But having received their diploma many have gone on to join the School's Advanced Study Group, where they attend regular seminars to learn osteopathic manipulations and chiropractic adjustments, herbalism and homeopathy. Now they can complete a special course in Applied Acupuncture under the aegis of the College of Acupuncture in London.

Some of these new manipulative therapists are highly critical of the osteopaths who do not use other therapies, and of the physiotherapists. 'If the osteopath or physiotherapist just manipulates the lesion or subluxation he is in the long term doing his patients a disservice,' one of them told me.

'They might feel better after their manipulation, but before long the problem reasserts itself, and they have to continue going back for more treatment.'

He admitted that temporary relief was better than being in constant pain, but continued with his argument, 'Some osteopaths have a patient going to them with a back pain. They find a lesion, and manipulate it. The treatment can take as little as fifteen minutes. While the patient may feel better, it is bad physical medicine. The osteopath has made no attempt at a real diagnosis, and that can only be done by taking a full and careful case history, blood and urine tests, and where necessary obtaining X-ray plates.

'Nor do they investigate the psychological state of the patient, for if the patient is under stress, and it doesn't matter where the stress is coming from, either his home or work, the tension will cause the lesion to reappear. And that is why I feel so much of osteopathy and physiotherapy today is only a form of first aid.'

Another manipulative therapist who holds similar views is Mr Stan W. Duncombe of Coventry, a man who has lectured upon his subject in the United States, Germany, Spain and throughout the British Isles. He informed me, 'If the body is healthy it will heal itself after the adjustment. If not, the subluxation will come back again as the total body is not ready or strong enough to allow the healing.'

Leaving aside the merits of this argument and concentrating upon the therapeutic effects of physical medicine, Mr Duncombe, like many eclectic osteopaths and manipulative therapists, sees a considerable number of young childern in the course of a week, with ages ranging from a few weeks to a few years old. He accepts that the birth process, and the early weeks of life, can cause a lesion, and if this remains undetected and uncorrected by the time the boy or girl is eleven years old it can lead to pigeon-toes, knock-knees and asthma, and in girls a problem with conceiving.

'If you take a close look at the asthmatic or emphysemic they are usually round-shouldered and knock-kneed, with their toes pointing either inwards or outwards at an exaggerated angle,' a therapist explained. He then proceeded to demonstrate with a lady that if she turned her toes in it made her buttocks stick out, and if she hunched her shoulder she was unable to take a deep breath and breathe normally. The lady agreed it was impossible, and the therapist went on, 'Over a period of time this posture must affect the bronchial tubes, the lungs, creating inflammation, and triggering off various reactions.'

In May 1973, the British Naturopathic and Osteopathic Association urged the creation of a new osteopathic health service for children in primary and secondary schools, to prevent the pupils from suffering from conditions caused by bad posture.

In keeping with this request of the BNOA, a physical therapist said that if there was a lesion around the seventh dorsal vertebra affecting the efficient functioning of the pancreas from birth, it could be an important contributory factor in the origins of diabetes. He emphasized that it may not be the only cause of the disease, nor did he propose that manipulation alone would cure it, although he had repeatedly demonstrated it could help the diabetic.

To the uninitiated it may seem strange that osteopaths claim that people prone to headaches can be suffering from the effects of childbirth, a fall or bump when young, and that the headaches will continue until the original fault is rectified. One practitioner said prior to the BNOA announcement, 'It is good preventive medicine to have a child visit an osteopath for regular physical check-ups, in the same way that he goes to see his dentist.'

Thinking about headaches, I saw that many of us have instinctively recognized that they can be alleviated by other methods than aspirin, for it is common practice to massage the neck and shoulders to relieve them if the time is available. Therefore it seems to me that the idea is a sound one, and I asked what was the ideal age for a child to commence the regular examinations. The answer was they should begin when the baby was about eight months old, because the bones and general physical health of a child is such that lesions can be corrected easily and without discomfort.

The deeper my investigation went into physical medicine the more I was forced to the conclusion that it would be impossible to deal with the entire range of the work these therapists cover, as it extends from skin conditions, through migraine, to cardiac disturbances, rheumatism, and a whole series of anxiety states which are usually lumped together under the blanket term of 'nerves'.

As heart diseases claim a large number of victims each year in all the highly developed technological countries, and because anxiety-tension-stress conditions are reaching plague proportions, I made the arbitrary decision to spotlight those two in these pages, because they appear to be of concern to all.

Mr Sidney Rose-Neil told a group of students how, as an osteopath and naturopath, he saw cardiac problems arising.

As a vegetarian he commenced outlining the dietary factors: excessive eating of animal fats could lead to the circulatory system becoming clogged and putting a greater strain upon the heart, as it had to pump the blood that much harder to ensure it reached all the extremities of the body. He then proceeded to mention how patients under constant occupational, marital, social or psychological stress learned to tighten the muscles in the solar plexus to the point where the heart and lungs were pressed up in to more confined space, putting a strain upon both organs, and preventing full chest expansion. This, he postulated, was the cause of certain heart and lung diseases.

Finally he mentioned osteopathic cardiology, and the ways in which spinal lesions or subluxations could have the same results as a 'muscle-bound' solar plexus. In the thesis he wrote for his

Doctorate in Osteopathy in July 1966, he provided case histories to show how combined osteopathic and naturopathic medicine, coupled with relaxation, had helped many suffering from functional hypertension.

Among his documented cases was that of a 62-year-old woman whose blood pressure was 230 over 130 when she went to him as a patient in September 1962. He ascertained that she was under constant emotional stress due to her husband being ill, and none of the drugs formerly prescribed for her had worked.

Mr Rose-Neil put her on a full naturopathic regime and saw her nine times, the first being on 9 September 1962, and the last on 20 December, 1962. During the four months he was treating her the blood pressure came down to 134 over 86, and at subsequent check-ups in 1965 and 1966 there had been no return of the previous symptomatology, and the blood pressure was 140/88 and 138/86 respectively.

His evidence was most convincing, but perhaps the idea that physical manipulation can be used in the treatment of neurosis and phobias is more startling and requires further explanation, because in the past it has been generally accepted that these were mental as opposed to physical manifestations.

To support the physical therapists' claim, there are some psychiatrists in the United States, and a few therapists I have personally trained in the United Kingdom, who do accept that *some* anxiety states, which Professor Sigmund Freud designated as being 'free-floating anxiety' and 'phobias', may indeed be rooted in the body.

Freud used the term 'free-floating anxiety' to cover those people who are in a constant state of apprehension without knowing what they are worrying about, and he proffered as the etiology of this type of anxiety the hypothesis that the worrier with these symptoms had, in the past, repressed into the unconscious mind incidents and feelings which were unacceptable to him at a conscious level. In other words he had experienced things he would rather forget, but the feelings of what he had experienced remained in the unconscious, bubbling away in an effort to obtain release. Although his explanation has been shown to be correct in specific cases, modern, non-Freudian psychiatrists in the United States have presented another explanation which, through their work, has proved to be equally valid.

According to them the physical symptoms of anxiety are a part of our human make-up, and are built into everyone for self-preservation. Collectively they are called 'the fight or flight mechanism', and become operative when anyone is threatened with a real or psychological threat situation.

When man was at his primitive stage of human development the mechanism was very useful. Then, if he came face to face with a ferocious animal he would perceive the threat through his senses, usually visually, and when the alarm signal was transmitted to the brain, the brain would prepare the body for action by tensing up the musculature, making the heart pump faster ready for action (palpitations), pumping adrenalin into the system, and attempting to empty the body of excessive weight by causing desire to urinate and/or defecate. Once this automatic procedure had been carried out man was mentally and physically in a state of readiness to fight the animal or to flee as fast as he could from it.

Today in the developed nations man no longer meets vicious predators stalking the streets of the towns and cities, if we discount the threat emanating from the modern animal – the mugger – but man still has the same self-preservation system working inside him.

Whenever man or woman faces a physical threat to security, and it could be an accident, the fear of being involved in a fight that has broken out, or anything else, the 'fight or flight mechanism' is activated, and there is exactly the same physical response when man or woman faces a psychological threat to security, the fear of losing a job, losing wife or lover . . .

But once the threat has passed over, the body relaxes, and this is where the new psychosomatic therapist believes the trouble lies. For it takes time for the body to relax, and if a person faces a series of real or psychological threats too quickly the body never has the opportunity to fully relax again, and the residue of tension left undischarged after each threat builds up until the body remains in a permanent state of fight or flight tension-readiness, although there is no real or psychological reason for it – a typical example of free-floating anxiety.

If the tension continues to build up after this point has been reached, the body sends its signal of alarm-readiness to the brain, and then the brain is in a quandary. The eyes and the other senses cannot detect any visible threat, and the mind cannot locate any psychological threat; hence the brain has to create something to fix the fear upon, as it is unable to function if the anomaly remains. It may create a fear of heights, fear of open spaces, fear of being in a confined space, fear of germs, blood, people, crowds . . .

According to the osteopaths, constant physical stress can cause subluxations to develop, and if that happens it becomes even more of a vicious circle. If a patient tries to relax the subluxations can prevent it, and if the attempt to relax persists pain appears in the affected area, and the discomfort causes the body to become rigid again in an effort to minimize it.

The American psychiatrists taking this new approach advocate teaching the patients the art of complete physical relaxation,[2] or using techniques to get the patients to re-enact the tension-provoking incidents and thus allowing the body to become tension-free.[3] Both groups then claim the anxiety states and phobias will remit, and they will quote their successful case histories to substantiate their particular therapeutic methodology.

That is logical, the physical therapists admit, but they maintain it can only be superficial unless the psychiatrists involved study physical medicine to allow them to conduct an osteopathic examination prior to commencing their particular programmes, because, if there are any undetected lesions or subluxations, whatever they attempt will be doomed.

Here controversy raises its head, and rather than become involved in the pros and the cons of the argument, for each faction has something to contribute, it is of more interest to close this survey of osteopathy by looking at the merits of the assertion made by some manipulative therapists that they can help infertile women to conceive, and assist men with a low sperm-count to become more procreative.

During my travels I met a gentleman who talked about the

large number of men and women who had been to see him with problems of infertility. The women, he assured me, had all been thoroughly examined by gynaecologists and told there was no organic reason for their infertility. Some of them had their fallopian tubes cleared to make conception easier, but all had remained barren. The men too had been through the orthodox procedures without any success. He conducted an examination of all of them, and in both men and women he found they had displaced pelvises. When he corrected the pelvic tilt his records showed that the women shortly afterwards became pregnant, while the former low sperm-count men found that their wives conceived.

He was naturally pleased with his success in this field, as were his patients, but there could be another explanation, which I put to him.

Everyone has met, or heard of, a lady who has wanted a child and after years of waiting has decided to wait no longer and adopt a son or daughter, only to find a few months later that she was pregnant.

There is a good psychological explanation for this pheno-menon. The woman could have had an unconscious fear of motherhood, wondering if she could cope with a child, and the unconscious fear could have brought about a state of physical tension which made her menstruate at the end of every month even if conception had been achieved earlier. As her desire to conceive became more important to her with the passage of time, physical stress built up during sexual intercourse as one thought was always present: 'Will I conceive this time?', and the tension-stress made the chances of conception even more remote. However, once the adoption had been completed, and the unconscious fears found to be without foundation, the woman relaxed, allowing nature to play its rightful role.

The same applies to men. When they are under stress, irrespective of the reason for it, they may well be adjudged fertile after a sperm count, but the tension-stress prevents them from impregnating their wives.

After listening to me patiently the therapist agreed that psychological reasons could play a part in apparent infertility. He also agreed that it was quite probable that the physical tension which the unconscious fears evoked might cause spinal displacements. But he continued: 'If the mind can cause physical reactions which prevent pregnancy, and we are agreed upon that, then, Peter, you will have to agree that if a patient has a fall, is in an accident, undergoes physical trauma in any form, then the resulting misalignment can have the same outcome, what you have referred to as apparent sterility.' To that there was no answer. In fact his line of argument impressed me to such a degree that it reinforced my earlier conclusion that by limiting my own work to psychotherapy, as I had done in the past, I had been denying my clients the complete therapy which they were entitled to expect; and that in future it would have to be combined with a type of physical therapy. For if it is accepted that the mind can affect the body, it is only logical that the body must influence the mind, and it may well be that before any illness is treated the practitioner, whether orthodox or heterodox, should begin by examining the back to see if there are any spinal displacements, before doing anything else.

Chiropractic - The Hand Medicine

While osteopathy is well known and accepted in Britain by the general public, if not by all members of the orthodox medical profession, the work of the chiropractor remains largely unknown. The few doctors whom I asked for their opinion of chiropractic medicine admitted they had no idea what I was talking about, and this is surprising as it is the branch of medicine that has grown more rapidly than any other medical speciality, with tens of thousands of Doctors of Chiropractic, DCs, now working in the United States, Canada, Australia, Switzerland, and throughout the world.

Even here in Britain there are approximately sixty qualified Doctors of Chiropractic without including many more manipulative therapists using chiropractic adjustments. And this situation is bound to alter before long as the Anglo-European College of Chiropractic, founded in 1965 in the south-coast seaside resort of Bournemouth, has students from all the European continental countries, the United States and Canada, plus an increasing number of British students undergoing a four-year training programme leading to their chiropractic doctorate. And some of the British students have received financial grants from their local education authorities to pay for the course.

Why are Americans and Canadians coming to the British College when they have Colleges of Chiropractic in their own countries? I put this question to a tutor at Anglo-European. He told me that it was happening because the American and Canadian establishments simply could not cope with the number of students wishing to become chiropractors, and therefore would-be students had to travel far afield if they wished to take the course in the immediate future.

This was interesting because it gives an insight into the rapid growth of chiropractic, but it raised a further question: 'How do chiropractors get their patients, since registered medical practitioners don't refer patients to them?'

The same tutor said that patients usually heard about chiropractic from a friend who had benefited from the treatment, and having got no relief from orthodox practitioners decided to see if the chiropractor could help them. When they arrived at the office the chiropractor would make a careful examination of the spine by means of X-ray, and possibly with a second diagnostic instrument the chiropractors have developed which detects spinal abnormalities by registering different heat temperatures. They also make a careful note of how the patient moves the body.

If the initial consultation reveals a displacement of the vertebra the patient is accepted for treatment, and the spinal anomalies corrected by a thrusting hand adjustment.

When patients obtain relief, and begin to understand the theory underlying chiropractic medicine, other members of the same family begin to see the chiropractor in the same role as the allopathic family physician, going to him for a number of clinical conditions which they previously thought were beyond the chiropractor's realm of competence. For even those who have scant knowledge of the work done by the chiropractor are apt to consider him as a glorified osteopath specializing in the usual back disorders, such as the so-called slipped disc, sciatica, lumbago, arthritis, frozen shoulder, etc.

The underlying theory of the system goes back to the time of its founder, Daniel David Palmer, a Canadian living in Davenport, Iowa, who it is claimed 'rediscovered' the art of hand medicine in 1895, when he was fifty years old.

Palmer had been interested in healing for a number of years, and the one thing which intrigued him more than anything else was why one person became ill and another didn't, and why one individual would get typhoid and another rheumatism. In his attempt to find an answer to this age-old riddle he studied osteopathy, which had been discovered by Dr Still in 1874. He thought it was an advance on orthodox medicine, but he could not accept the osteopathic concept of the free flow of blood, and he therefore chose to work as a 'magnetic healer', as a follower of Dr Franz Anton Mesmer. Yet it is obvious that his earlier study of the infant science of osteopathy stood him in good stead when, on 18 September 1895, the long arm of coincidence reached out to him in the form of his office janitor, Harvey Lillard, who was deaf.

Upon being questioned about how his deafness happened, Mr Lillard told Palmer how, seventeen years earlier, he had stooped down when he was working and felt something happen to his back. From that moment on he became deaf.

And it was at that juncture, I feel sure, that Palmer's earlier investigation of osteopathy came back to him in the form of a hunch, encouraging him to examine the spine to see if there was any abnormality which could have played a part in Lillard's deafness. He found what his intuition had suggested, a displaced vertebra, and the janitor confirmed that it was that exact spot which had hurt him at the time he lost his hearing. Palmer then allowed his intuition to guide him further. Using a short thrust with his hand he literally shot the vertebra back into position, and shortly afterwards Lillard's hearing returned to normal.

On that day, and on that occasion D. D. Palmer had discovered a therapy, and his next step was to search for a theory to explain how it worked, because work it did, as people came to him from many places and all walks of life when the news of what he was doing reached them.

Doing his homework well, Palmer arrived at the conclusion that when any part of the spine is dislocated, irrespective of the cause of the dislocation, the nerves leading from the backbone are trapped and prevented from transmitting the appropriate healthy signals from the brain to the organ or organs involved, and vice versa. Taking his theory further he maintained that as time passes the trapped nerve causes an irritation, poisons begin to accumulate, and illness is the result. In his book *The Science and Art and Philosophy of Chiropractic*,[1] Palmer urged that 'Students of Chiropractic should constantly remember that

disease is not a thing, but a *condition*. It is an *abnormal* performance of certain morphological alterations of the body; agencies
and conditions which the body cannot adapt itself to, sway
the capacities of energy above or below normal, inducing
the *functional aberrations* and structural alternations known as
disease.

'The science of chiropractic has modified our views concerning life, death, health and disease. We no longer believe that
disease is an entity, something foreign to the body, which may
enter from without, and with which we have to grasp, struggle,
fight and conquer, or submit and succumb to its ravages. Disease
is a disturbed condition, not a thing or entity. Disease is an
abnormal performance of certain functions; the abnormal activity
has its causes.'

Perhaps owing to modesty or to give his method of treatment
an aura of tradition and age, Palmer made no claims to have discovered a new form of medicine, rather he suggested he had
rediscovered a healing art which had been used long ago and
which had been lost in the intervening years. Accordingly, when
one of his earlier satisfied patients, the Reverend Samuel Weed,
turned out to be a Greek scholar, Palmer asked the Reverend
Weed if there was a Greek word meaning 'done by hand'. Weed
said there was: *cheir* (hand) and *praktikos* (practitioner); hence
the term chiropractor – Hand Practitioner.

In support of his founder's claim to antiquity the modern
chiropractor is apt to quote from a book by Dr K. A. Ligeros,
MD, PhD, of Athens, Greece, entitled, *How Ancient Healing
Governs Modern Therapeutics*.

The frontispiece of Ligeros' book is a photograph of an ancient
carving from the fifth century BC showing a manipulative adjustment of the upper dorsal spine being carried out, and on page
420 the Greek doctor refers to the Father of Medicine, Hippocrates (460–370 BC), in these words: 'Hippocrates more than
once called the attention of the practitioner to these truths,
admonishing him, as well as the prospective student, to endeavour to learn to comprehend well the nature of the spinal column,
to study closely its structure and, so to say, functions. Such
study, he advised, is necessary in many diseases.'

On the same page of the book Hippocrates is quoted further: 'One or more vertebrae of the spine may or may not go out of place very much' or 'they might give way very little, and if they do, they are likely to produce serious complications and even death, if not properly adjusted.'[2]

Once the philosophy and practice of chiropractic are understood they explain how and why chiropractors maintain that they can treat conditions which the orthodox practitioner would consider to be organic and outside the area of manipulative therapy. But there is an adage: 'The proof of the pudding is in the eating.'

Apart from individual case histories, the proof that chiropractic is as successful as allopathic in some illnesses, and better in others, comes from two primary sources.

As many insurance companies in the United States recognize the value of this modality, and members of health insurance programmes can receive treatment from a chiropractor under the various schemes, the Insurance Relations Committee of the Florida Chiropractic Association did an analysis of all cases of industrial sprains and strains of the neck and back occurring in Florida in 1956, and had its findings of the 19,666 cases checked by an independent research body, the First Research Corporation.

A summary of the findings provided the following information: 'In sprain and strain cases handled by physicians, the treatment costs were 27.5 per cent higher than in those treated by a chiropractor.

'Compensation costs under a physician's care averaged 311 per cent more . . .

'Average time lost from work by the patient was three days under chiropractic care, compared with nine days under a physician's care. When under the care of a medical specialist, the patient lost 30 days from work, compared with 2.5 under chiropractic care.'[3]

If we look at these figures, and the time saved away from work, it is not surprising that a number of companies both in the US and Britain are now employing chiropractors, or manipulative therapists with knowledge of chiropractic adjustments, to look after the needs of their staff by holding regular clinics at their factories.

The second source comes from Denmark, where the Danish government is considering the integration of chiropractic into the State Health Insurance Scheme when the service is expanded this year (1973), and can be found in the British Pro-Chiropractic Bulletin.

In the bulletin a favourable Danish government report is quoted as saying, among other things:

> the majority [of the committee] is of the opinion that the chiro-practic method of treatment on the spine and pelvis, is so defined and so well exercised by chiropractors, who have learned this method of treatment in the Colleges acknowledged by the Danish Chiropractors Council,[4] that it should be considered if a way can be found to incorporate this manner of treatment in the Danish medical and social laws in such a way that the Sick-Insurance Benefit Scheme and Private Sick-Insurance Associations fully or in part can cover the costs of such treat-ment for members.

The Copenhagen County Council states that, in the Physio-therapeutic Department of the County Hospital, every patient-day costs £21. On the average each patient is hospitalized for twelve days at an approximate cost of £225.

The Ministry of the Interior has assembled statistical infor-mation on chiropractic treatment in chiropractic practices and clinics and states that the cost of examining a patient, X-ray, and the average number of treatments is £17 – the saving is therefore £238 per patient.

The ministry states that from a study of 1,024 chiropractic patient case histories it is considered that 521 would have been sent by physicians to the Hospital Physio-therapeutic Depart-ment for treatment there. For these the total cost of hospital treatment would have been £132,850.

Statistical analyses conducted by the Ministry lead to con-clusions that about 30,000 chiropractic patients are given treatment annually in Denmark. After applying a complicated 'profit and loss' adjustment for differing types of cases it is estimated that, but for the availability of chiropractic treatment, the cost of treating these cases would have been at least an additional £5 million.

Savings in lost working days, lost wages and sick insurance benefit refunds cannot be calculated from the materials available in this statistical survey.[5]

While this evidence is impressive it relates to sprains and strains, whereas D. D. Palmer and later chiropractors have been emphatic about their ability to treat a far wider range of illnesses. This is why I was pleased when Dr John R. Denton, DC, a lecturer at the Anglo-European College of Chiropractic, gave me a number of individual case histories to show the diversity of conditions that can respond to treatment.

He prefaced the material he was going to give me by explaining that their yardstick for accepting a person as a patient did not depend upon the presenting symptom. They considered that a disturbance of the nervous system was behind most pathologies to some degree, and that therefore if a patient had a spinal abnormality they would accept him or her, and if there was no spinal displacement they would recommend the patient to go elsewhere.

The first case history I was given related to an eleven-year-old boy who had been suffering from bronchial asthma since birth. He had one minor attack of asthma shortly after commencing chiropractic treatment, but that was to be his last, and he went through the following winter free from attacks, whereas formerly he had suffered an attack once a week.

As Dr Denton told me about the boy I was reminded of how closely chiropractic resembled the Chinese form of medicine, acupuncture, because they both appeared to have similiar ideas about illness. Their treatment may be different but it was the similarity which reminded me of a conversation which a leading British acupuncturist in Liverpool had had with my partner, Tony Dickenson. The acupuncturist said he had made a study of some 200 bronchial asthmatics who had been in treatment with him, and out of those he had obtained ninety per cent remission. Tony then asked him what his success rate was with functional asthma, and he was told the results were by no means as good. This was of interest to both of us as we had found in cases of functional asthma that hypno-analysis and hypnotic symptom control was helpful in more than eighty per cent of the people we saw, but we had a poor success rate with bronchial asthma.

A female patient went to the College's clinic with high blood pressure and complaining of vertigo. The blood pressure was quickly restored to normal for her age and the accompanying vertigo disappeared. In this instance I was not over-impressed as I was aware that a patient who suffers from anxiety can often have attacks of vertigo. Therefore it need not have been the chiropractic adjustment which brought about the remission, but the fact that something positive was being done to help her, together with her faith in the practitioner. I put my doubts in the form of a question to Dr Denton: 'How much, in a case like this, could the healing process have been set in motion because she had faith in you as a chiropractor, so that the cure was as much due to her personal committal to you as to the actual therapy?'

Dr Denton agreed that this aspect of healing had always to be taken into consideration, whether the practitioner was a registered doctor or a witchdoctor, 'But in her case the commitment was minimal as the woman came in very sceptical indeed, and got better almost in spite of herself.'

He added that chiropractors were often accused of treating psychosomatic conditions, 'But it is interesting how they only become that after they were failures of medicine.'

Another case history given to me referred to a young woman who had a more-or-less permanent backache in the lumbar region, high blood pressure, suffered from anxiety and periodic severe depression, and had immense problems at the times of menstruation. All her symptoms appeared when she first began to menstruate at the age of thirteen, and proved to be resistant to all forms of orthodox medicine which had been tried prior to her going to the College. Upon chiropractic examination it was found there was a subluxation in the lumbar region which responded to adjustment, and all the symptomatology completely remitted as a result.

We also discussed how chiropractic could assist cases of anxiety, and in confirmation of this I was given a copy of the medical weekly, *General Practitioner,* which showed how anxiety and depression could be caused by cervical displacement and pressure.[6] The author of the article, Dr Ebbetts, said that in those cases where it is diagnosed that there is cervical joint trauma accompanying the anxiety-depression, the treatment is comparatively simple and can be learned by a doctor in a short time. This observation wasn't new to the chiropractors as they had long ago discovered that adjustment could relieve many cases of depression as quickly and more permanently than pharmaceutical anti-depressants, and a Doctor of Chiropractic informed me: 'Where we find there are specific spinal lesions, particularly in the cervical regions, these do affect the person's mental outlook . . . and once we work on these, the lesions, it breaks the circle of depression at that point.'

My interviews at the College and with other chiropractors could have been interminable, but it was in a book, *The Foundation of Chiropractic from the Standpoint of a Physician,* written by Dr Freimut Biedermann, MD, of Stuttgart, that there was a list of responding conditions which is so vast that it causes many chiropractors to blush. These included arthritis obliterans, haemorrhoids, impotence, intermittent claudication, menstrual disturbance, tetany, toothache, urethritis, gall-bladder colic, renal colic, paroxysmal vomiting, allergic manifestations, etc.

But, in spite of all the evidence, and discounting a proportion of it because of the enthusiasm of the chiropractors, the orthodox medical profession prefers to ignore chiropractic. The few allopathic practitioners who believe it may have something to contribute consider it as another type of pill they can add to their list, as a technique that can be mastered in a few weekend demonstration-teaching seminars, and believe that its use should be confined to registered medical practitioners.

In the United States there is a bitter feud being waged between the chiropractors and the American Medical Association. Although Doctors of Chiropractic are licensed to practise in many States of the Union this does not mean to say they are accepted, as the 'National Congress on Medical Quackery', held in Washington, DC, in October 1961, revealed. Those attending the congress sponsored by the AMA and the Food and Drug Administration were told by Mr Oliver Field, Director of the American Medical Associations Department of Investigation, that he recommended a programme be launched to discourage young people from entering chiropractic colleges and schools. Mr Field further charged the Federal US Government with sponsoring and spawning quackery by providing military veterans with money to attend such schools.

Writing in his Brief to the Canadian Royal Commission on Health Services in 1962, Dr D. C. Sutherland, DC, made the pertinent comment: 'It would appear that the methods [chiropractic] are acceptable only when under complete medical domination and control.' Later Dr Sutherland said that the General Practitioner, 'untrained and unskilled in the art of spinal adjusting, is being advised empirically to experiment in these skilled procedures.' Giving his justification for claiming that registered practitioners are being misled, he referred to the article 'The Simple Problems of Backache' by Dr Gerald L. Burke, MD, of Vancouver, BC, in which Dr Burke suggests 'that the physician practise a few times on his wife or colleague to demonstrate that though obviously great force is applied through leverage, not the slightest harm will be done.' Dr Sutherland said, 'We strongly suggest that advice such as this is highly improper and certainly not in the best interests of the public welfare.'

Neither is the struggle between the orthodox and heterodox schools of medical thought in the best interests of the patient, and the orthodox attitude is unnecessary because the chiropractors do not want to become a part of the orthodox system. On the contrary, they want to be accepted as having something to offer certain patients, and not to be incorporated into orthodox ranks as they see that as being the first step in their eventual demise. Their viewpoint on this was clearly expressed by Dr A. E. Homewood, DC, the Dean of the Canadian Memorial Chiropractic College of Toronto, Canada, writing in an issue of the University of Toronto Medical Journal,[7] when he informed orthodox medical students that after homeopathy was accepted into the orthodox fold it became virtually extinct.

'The osteopaths sought and found favour with allopathic medicine at the expense of the manipulative art. Hence, to have chiropractic accepted into the orthodox fold, to become a part of medicine, or to be given the privileges of practising general medicine as well as manipulation, would lead to a loss of this art. There is room in the healing arts for a number of schools of thought . . . Were a single school of healing to exist, the sick would be the losers, and the incentive for progress would be seriously dulled.'

11

Secrets of the Body

Over the years I have been using hypnosis and hypno-analysis to help people overcome anxiety, tension and stress in its varied symptomatic forms. I have occasionally met the client who has failed to respond although I felt he or she should have done. Of course this is not unusual. It is universally recognized that in all forms of medicine and therapy, irrespective of how good the therapist is, failures will occur from time to time, and students are taught that this is unfortunate but also unavoidable.

At a superficial level I could accept this happening. I knew that a doctor will treat thousands of patients suffering from an illness and they will all recover, bar one. In that instance the autopsy would reveal the cause of death, but it would rarely clarify why that one patient out of all the preceding thousands should die. And it was that question mark, the 'why', which forced me to examine and re-examine my own therapeutic procedures to try and locate what I had overlooked in the course of my work.

The clients I worked with were all suitable for hypnotherapy. In each and every case I used the hypno-diagnostic process to ensure that the unconscious mind of the client determined the approach which was best for them, instead of relying upon my own experience and giving them what I considered to be correct.[1]

When hypno-analysis was indicated I would assist the client to trace back over the years and to recall the long forgotten events which led up to the actual appearance of the symptomatology. After each analytic session we would discuss the implications of the materials and memories we had uncovered, and finally to conclude the course of treatment I would use a type of Reality Therapy in the form of hypnotic suggestions to help each client cope with life in future without anxiety.

Admittedly in most cases this worked, but why not in all of them?

It would have been easy to dismiss my failures with excuses: 'Their home or work situation continued to aggravate the condition, and as I could not alter those situations their symptoms were bound to continue'; or 'They didn't really want to get well,' because as a famous teaching psychiatrist used to tell his students, 'If you could shoot the father, the mother, the brother or sister, the husband or wife at the appropriate moment in time then you would be able to cure all those who will come to you seeking your aid.'

I could not take that easy way out so my search for an answer went on. My friends assured me my searching was pointless and suggested that I grow up, as according to their reasoning my inability to face my own limitations was a sign of immaturity, and I had to learn to accept ego-deflation whenever I failed. They may have been correct in their assessment of me, but I still had to go on.

The first glimmer of light came to me a number of years ago when I read the work of the late Dr Wilhelm Reich, MD, and learned that he had faced a similar dilemma. He discovered that people developed a 'character armour' to protect themselves, or, put more simply, Reich came to the conclusion that we mirrored our neuroses in our bodies, and there is a definite *Body Language* which the psychotherapist and psychoanalyst has to understand.

The man who holds back what he would really like to say to other people learns to physically control himself by keeping his mouth tightly shut, his teeth and jaws tightly clenched, and before long he forgets what he wanted to say as it is firmly buried behind the 'character armour' of his mouth and jaws. If he undergoes psychoanalysis he will prove to be resistant, because his mouth and jaws will prevent him from recalling and telling the analyst what he originally wanted to say.

The person who is frightened of recognizing his or her own

body feelings in certain situations will tighten up the muscles in the solar plexus, the abdomen, and soon find themselves holding their bodies in an upright, permanently tensed position.

According to Reich all of us have learned how to control and inhibit our emotions by armouring up the appropriate parts of our bodies. Some of us have done it better than others, but it is the body character armour which is the final neurotic defence, and unless the armour is dispersed psychotherapy will be unsuccessful.[2]

Having isolated the problem Reich developed therapeutic procedures to loosen the character armour, and other psychiatrists, psychotherapists and psychologists have steadily taken his work further – people like Trygve Braaty, who discovered that certain people undergoing physiotherapy would abreact (relive) traumatic episodes from their past which had previously been bound up in their muscular rigidity;[3] Dr Alexander Lowen, MD, of New York City, who founded the Institute of Bio-Energetic Analysis, added more information to show how tension could become bound up in the body, and worked out his own techniques for releasing the blocked-up energy;[4] Dr Arthur Janov of Los Angeles more recently developed his way of releasing the character armour through Primal Therapy,[5] and after them the list becomes endless.

As far as my own problem with hypno- and psycho-therapy were concerned the work of Reich and the neo-Reichians was a step forward in the right direction, and I began to combine some of their techniques into my own therapeutic approach. But they still appeared to me to be too cumbersome, and hit-and-miss, although I am sure that Drs Lowen and Janov would heartily disagree with me on this.

Then came a partial breakthrough.

An Israeli Doctor of Acupuncture and a Manipulative Therapist, Giora Harel, telephoned me to say that while he was manipulating the body of a patient he had found that if he relaxed the patient for an hour or more the patient still retained tension in a specific part of the body. He had instinctively applied heavy pressure with one of his fingers to the centre of the remaining tension, and he found it moved to another part of the body.

Then it moved again, and continued to jump from one area to another until it appeared to reach the source of the physical tension, and when that happened the patient abreacted – re-enacted and relived – a painful episode from his or her past; the musculature relaxed and the tension temporarily disappeared. He informed me that by repeating this until the body was completely free from tension he had managed to help patients who had been resistant to other types of psychotherapy.

Before he put the telephone down he said he was going to demonstrate his findings to a small group of practitioners in London, and if I would like to attend he would be pleased to have me in the group as an observer. It was too good an opportunity to miss.

The acupuncturist told all of us who had assembled at his seminar how he had made his discovery, after which he proceeded to demonstrate what he did on a young lady. Perhaps it was because there were observers present in the room, but while her body did eventually go into an uncontrollable convulsion and she began sobbing, resulting in her admitting she felt much better after it had subsided, the demonstration did not live up to the claims Giora Harel had made for it. But I was sure from what I had witnessed that the case histories he had presented, together with details of patients' reactions, had happened under more conducive conditions.

We had an opportunity to talk before I started driving back to the north of England.

I told Harel I had been impressed, although I added the proviso that the technique as he had presented it took far too long, was still hit-or-miss, and needed a lot more practical research and refining before it could be considered as a valuable weapon in the armoury against anxiety states.

'That is why I asked you to be here,' he said. 'There must be a way of combining your own hypnotic diagnostic and hypnotic analytical approach to it so that it becomes really effective. Do you think you can do it?'

To escape from having to commit myself I replied, 'Giora, leave it with me for a time, and I will see what I can come up with.'

When I got back home my students who knew why I had gone down to London asked me to give them a resumé, and most of them were excited by the possibilities it offered. They asked if we could have an actual working session to see what happened to them.

I agreed. Time was scheduled for the experiment, and we went ahead, but again it was only partially successful.

Some students taking part found it released a lot of their tension, and one of them found her tension traversed through the body until it moved into her left arm, then into her little finger, and as the tension apparently flowed out into thin air she burst into a paroxysm of uncontrolled sobbing. She said she felt better after all the tears had been spent, and from the peaceful look on her face the group concluded it had been more beneficial for her than for any of them.

After that brief incursion into body-tension release the entire concept lay dormant for a while; that is, until I had to go to the Tyringham Naturopathic Clinic to see Mr Sidney Rose-Neil about some other research I was doing.

When our work was concluded Mr Rose-Neil and I were sitting in the lounge of his home talking about things in general when I mentioned the Harel concept, and what had happened with the students. Immediately Sidney became alert.

'Didn't you know I did a lot of work in a similiar field as long ago as the mid-1950s?' he asked.

I acknowledged my ignorance.

'Yes, I did a thesis in July 1966, entitled, "The Treatment of Neuro-muscular Spasm by Co-ordinated Therapy of Relaxation, Neuro-muscular and Osteopathic Manipulation, and its Related Extension to Functional Hypertension" – quite a mouthful – but in it I related some of my findings. I will lend you a copy of the thesis if you wish.'

What he had done was not exactly the same, but he showed from a collection of case histories how a combination of relaxation and osteopathic manipulation had provided long-sought-for relief.

A typical example was a thirty-one-year-old schoolteacher who consulted him in September 1957, with pain in the cervical area of the spine, insomnia, constipation and dysmenorrhea. She had been seeing her own osteopath where she lived, but without any long-lasting result. Rose-Neil commenced his combined relaxation and manipulative therapy in September 1957 and the patient was discharged, free from symptoms, in February 1958; and there was no relapse during the following eight years.

Mr Rose-Neil also commented: 'I have found a number of my own patients abreacting while I have been using relaxation and manipulation, but I have tried to stem the outbursts. From what you have said I now see that I should have encouraged them rather than trying to get the patients to repress their emotions.'

Our parting agreement was that we would keep in contact, and I would try developing the theme further.

The final breakthrough came with a client I had had in therapy but still found she had strong physical tension in a specific body area even when we had gone through the hypnotic relaxation procedure. Previously I would have accepted that as being transitory, something which would recede as the hypnotic relaxation became familiar to her. However, on this occasion I decided to ask her unconscious mind whether the physical tension was related to her presenting symptoms.

In order that the reader may follow what happened I will explain how contact with the unconscious mind is made in hypno-diagnosis.

With all the clients I see I establish an ideo-motor, involuntary, control of the index finger of the left hand in this way:

> In a few seconds time, when I say the word 'Now', your unconscious mind is taking control of the first finger of your left hand, and without any conscious effort on your part whatsoever your unconscious mind is making the first finger of your left hand very, very light. In fact the first finger of your left hand is so light that the first finger of your left hand is lifting up off the arm of the chair, and continuing to lift up until I ask it to stop . . .

After inducing hypnosis I established the ideo-motor signal with the lady in question, and said to her:

You have told me that you still have this tension in your back, and what we both need to know is if the physical tension is directly related to the problem you have been having. Now, you would not consciously know the answer to that question, but I believe that your unconscious mind, which knows everything about you, will be able to give us the answer. That being the case, when I say the word 'tension' in a few seconds time, if the remaining physical tension is a part of your problem and needs to be investigated before we proceed further with our usual therapy, your unconscious mind will know that it has to be investigated. And it is able to tell you and me that it is necessary by lifting up the first finger of your left hand very quickly and very high when I say the word 'tension' in a few seconds time. On the other hand if the remaining physical tension is not directly related to your problem, your unconscious mind will know that too, and if it is not directly linked it will be able to tell us by leaving the first finger of your left hand perfectly still irrespective of what I may say. So ready, 'tension'.

The first finger lifted up quickly, confirming the tension's relevance to her problem, and having obtained confirmation I went on to what I considered to be the next step. I told her that I was going to find the *core,* the centre of the tension by applying finger pressure to the general area of the tension, asking her to tell me when I had located the most painful or tender spot. This took a matter of seconds.

Good! Now we have located the core of the tension, and as I keep my finger on the same spot all the time you will find the tension building up under it until it becomes very pronounced, then, when it cannot get any stronger the tension will move to another part of the body. When it moves I want you to tell me exactly where it has moved to, and before long, and quite quickly the tension will go to that part of the body where it really belongs. Then, and only when the tension has gone to the part of your body where it really belongs and has its origins, will the first finger of your left hand lift up to let me know that the tension will not move again: that we have located the original spot of the tension, and can proceed from there.

The tension moved to various parts of her body as we traced it back to the beginning, and it finally settled in the upper part of her chest.

I congratulated her on our progress, adding:

As we have now found the real source of the tension our next step is to find out what the tension means and what caused it, and this is how we are going to do it. In a few seconds time I am going to say the word 'origin' and when I say the word 'origin', each time I repeat it the tension is mounting in intensity until it quickly reaches the stage where you can no longer contain it. At that moment you will know exactly what the tension means. You will remember, recall or relive exactly what caused the tension to be here, and it will burst out in words and emotion, in fact in any way necessary for you to rid yourself of the tension . . .

With her the cause was repressed anger and frustration stemming from an incident in her early childhood, an incident where she had been unfairly accused by her father of doing something 'naughty', and when she tried to explain to him what really happened her father kept on smacking her, telling her to keep quiet and stop telling him any more lies.

As her crying ceased and before we terminated the hypnosis she said, 'It is funny, but ever since I was a little girl I have never been able to exert my own personality. I have wanted to many times. I have wanted to say what I really thought, but I couldn't. I found myself always agreeing with what others said, and with what I felt others expected of me. I have always held myself back. I have never been able to be me. God, but I want to be me. Help me . . . Help me. . .'

It would be pleasant if I could write that this client was cured, whatever that word may mean, after the session. She wasn't. However, she felt more free in her body and psychologically than she could ever remember feeling, and at our subsequent sessions her body gave up more of its secrets so that eventually all aspects of her anxiety syndrome subsided. When she relaxed there was no trace of any lingering tension, and she was able to live normally for the first time in her life.[6]

From that moment I started to make this an integral part of my therapeutic routine, and I ask each client after they have relaxed into the so-called hypnotic state if they still have some physical tension remaining. If they have I commence working upon their muscular tensions before taking them into analysis, and to my surprise I have found that further hypno-analysis is often not necessary.

I have also used it on clients who had been in therapy with me and who were not making the progress we expected, and the results have been little short of remarkable.

My work had forced me to the conclusion that psychotherapists who deal solely with the psyche are doing their clients a disservice, and if psychotherapy and hypnosis are to have a role in modern medicine their therapists will need to look to the body with as much intensity as they had previously concentrated upon the mind. The same also applies to manipulative therapists who have no knowledge of the psyche. When I returned to Tyringham to discuss my views and findings with Sidney Rose-Neil he was in agreement with me and together we made plans for training seminars to be held at the Institute of Psychosomatic Therapy to teach the new therapy, which we decided to call Psycho-Muscular Release Therapy (PMRT).

Due to our individual commitments we were unable to put our plans into operation until later, so I continued working with PMRT, and conducting a few short courses in its application.

It was at one of the seminars I held in the south of England that a lady therapist volunteered to act as a guinea-pig for demonstration purposes. She informed the group she had constant tension in her back, and had been suffering from laryngitis for the past few weeks, which prevented her from talking properly, and it had not responded to orthodox treatment.

By the use of a rapid hypnotic induction technique which takes less than three minutes to apply, she entered the relaxed state of hypnosis, and the tension started out on a circuitous route before it ended up in her throat. Finger-pressure was maintained as the tension built up, and then the volunteer indicated she knew what the physical tension meant and how it had arisen. Five weeks earlier her son had been the cause of much concern to her, and there was a lot she wanted to tell him, but he too was very upset and she decided to say nothing.

I asked her if she still needed to hold the tension in her neck. Her answer was 'No', therefore I terminated the session, and, as she sat up on the massage plinth which I had been using, her voice was perfectly normal. There was no trace of the earlier laryngitis, and there was no ache in the back.

Another Psycho-Muscular Release Therapist worked with a lady in her late twenties who had a long history of anxiety disorders. At their initial consultation she complained of constant irritability leading to occasional irrational outbursts, a general feeling of personal dissatisfaction, and a tightness in the stomach which was always present and prevented her from relaxing. When her therapist suggested the rigidity in the stomach might have a psychological meaning she considered it to be ridiculous. She wanted hypno-analysis, and she was sure the constant tightness in her stomach resulted from her having had children, and from a need to keep her stomach pulled in to maintain her figure.

On the surface her explanation was most reasonable, but when she was in hypnosis the stomach tightness remained, and the ideo-motor signal gave a positive indication that it was a physical manifestation of a repression.

At their first real PMRT session the tightness-tension moved from her stomach into one hand and then into another, both locations having their own meaning. One was sexual, a fear she would initiate sexual advances to her husband, and this she felt guilty about as her mother had always instilled into her the idea that anything sexual was 'dirty'. The other meaning was that she had to keep the tension in her hand to prevent her from smacking her son.

Immediately following the session they talked about the fears lying behind the physical tension, and the patient confirmed she felt better, the tightness having gone from her stomach. But it returned, and at their next meeting it was traced out again, with each place it visited being investigated.

The further into therapy they got the more obvious it became to the therapist that the resistance to the actual genesis was manifesting itself by more rapid jumps from one part of the body to another – a good sign, as I had often found this heralded the final step in the treatment.

True to form, at the next meeting the crux of her problem was revealed.

The tightness was back in her stomach at the outset. Then it went into the vagina and stayed there. Bit by bit the therapist built up the tension inside the sexual orifice until it could no longer be contained. The explanation was that it had been necessary to protect herself from her own sexuality, because she felt she dare not be herself in case her true sexual self was unacceptable to her husband and to the other people she held in high esteem.

On that occasion, when the session was over, the client and therapist talked about what had emerged. She felt a new flow of energy in her body, just as if her body had come to life. Her former anxiety syndrome appeared to have gone. At the time of writing she had not had a relapse.

What has emerged from my own work with hypnotic PMRT, together with the findings of those therapists I have trained in its application, is that underlying an individual's character armouring is a denial of *self;* that the clients have been forced through circumstances in the past to bury their pain, anger, frustration, bitterness, etc., into their physical structure, and their repressed emotions – energy – have to be released before the client can make psychological adjustments to their life-style. A final case history will illustrate this.

An attractive lady in her early 40s came to see me, with constant pain in her back, together with a feeling of depressive sadness which she could not account for. She told me she had been to see both a chiropractor and an osteopath, but the relief obtained was only temporary.

At our first PMRT meeting she recognized that the tension, which traversed from her back to her chest, was a part of her sadness. She burst out crying and said it was related to something she really 'wanted to get off her chest'. I asked her what it was. There was a gentleman she knew who was continually placing her in an untenable position, and she had no idea how she could escape from the web he had spun around her. She wanted to get out; she did not like the position she was in, but she could not decide how to act because it would hurt her male friend.

In the course of our meeting five more times it became apparent she had reached a stage in her life when she wanted to be herself. Formerly she had had a professional occupation, but it had ceased to give her satisfaction, and she had decided to go into business for herself. And that is where she ran headlong into obstacles. Everyone seemed to thwart her at every turn in both her personal and business life. They all knew what was best for her, and expected her to follow their advice, even though it was contrary to her own wishes.

The feeling of being trapped and unable to live her own life was not new to her. She had known it for as long as she could remember, and the only reason why her internal conflicts had loomed up was because she had realized that if she didn't break out of the trap then, she would have to deny her individuality once and for all.

She knew what she wanted to do, but did not know how to carry out her plans without meeting overwhelming antagonism.

We discussed the alternatives open to her, and how best to approach them, and the feeling of conflict did remit for short periods, but the pain in her back kept on returning to exactly the same spot.

It was the sixth session that PMRT provided the answer. As the tension-pain built up inside her she faced its origin. It was migraine!

That was a shock to both of us, and it was a pity that she had failed to tell me that she had suffered from migraine for years, and had only been apparently cured of it by a manipulative therapist shortly before.

As the moment of final insight came the lady exclaimed, 'Of course, I know what it is now. I remember. I got this pain in my back as soon as the other therapist stopped the migraine attacks, but I have never linked the two together before now.'

It was a clear-cut example of symptom-transference, about which a lot is talked and written, yet it is rarely taken into consideration during therapy.

If I had known earlier that she had had a history of migraine I might have saved both of us time, because I had worked extensively with migraine and hypnosis and found that all my migrainous clients had an identical personality profile. They were all people who were unable to be themselves and release their emotions in any way whatsoever, and the migraine attacks afflicting them could be compared to a fountain of energy.

Because they had no natural outlet for their pent-up emotions/ energy, it built up inside them until it spilled over in the same way that a fountain does at the peak of its flow, affecting the head, the eyes and ultimately the stomach. My observations also take cognizance of the vascular factors, the forcing of blood into the brain and the restriction of the veins, because I see those as a part of inhibited energy.

People may disagree with my analysis of the migraine sufferer for that is their prerogative; nevertheless the remission of migraine symptoms without symptom-transference following hypno-analysis provides sufficient evidence to support my assertion, and if it were more generally recognized by orthodox and heterodox medical practitioners they would find they could assist their own migraine patients to a greater extent than at present.

But let me draw this part of the book to a close by putting on record that what I have discovered in hypnotic Psycho-Muscular Release Therapy is not new. Reich, Lowen and many others who have looked to the body for answers provided me with the background, as did Sigmund Freud, because as a young doctor he came across the muscular release syndrome but failed to see its significance in a therapeutic context.

The story behind Freud's oversight begins when he went to Paris in 1885 to study hysteria under the famous Professor Charcot at the Salpêtrière Hospital. As he made his rounds of the hospital's wards, and attended Charcot's lectures, he saw that many patients suffering from hysterical paralysis had what were then termed 'hysterogenic zones' – a part of their body which, when pressed, caused them to physically react in one way or another, including verbalization, and in certain instances paralyzed limbs were reactivated into positive movement.

The hysteric manifestations were dismissed as being nothing but interesting phenomena, whereas today's body-therapists of all the different disciplines see those former hysterogenic zones as buttons which can be pressed to release pent-up energy, thereby lowering the anxiety level bubbling away inside their patients and clients.

Nor are the hypnotic relaxation techniques I employ new, because relaxation has long been considered an essential part of the treatment for anxiety states, hence many out-patient psychiatric clinics hold relaxation classes to teach the patients the art of relaxation, and how to cope with their everyday lives in a more relaxed manner.

What I have done with Psycho-Muscular Release Therapy is to invert relaxation; to use it as a means of highlighting residual tension in order to understand its presence and disperse it. I also hope that I have managed to take hypnosis out of the nineteenth-century shadows, and given it a new and more vital role to play. But more important than all this, I hope the medical profession as a whole will see from PMRT that the body does contain and retain secrets which can be detrimental to the health and well-being of people, and that medical practitioners will have to become more aware of body-language, because it can show them the mental state of their patients.

12

The Future of Human Medicine

With the threat of iatrogenic illness hanging over the heads of an increasing number of people receiving chemotherapy for a variety of functional and organic disorders, coupled with the growing danger of people becoming dependent upon non-prescription drugs to treat all manner of minor ailments ranging from a headache at one end to constipation at the other, it is obvious that this situation cannot continue unabated. Nor does it require the services of a clairvoyant to foresee that the time is coming when those practising the science and art of medicine will have to re-orient their thinking and seek alternative methods of combating disease.

That the alternatives do exist and can work has been shown in the previous pages of this book, but the important question that has to be answered is: 'How will the drugless alternatives fit into a new medical system?'

Before a realistic answer can be formulated it is necessary to understand that the question touches upon two entirely separate problems.

The first of these is that as long as the orthodox medical establishment remains the supreme arbiter in matters medical, and governments continue to see orthodox medical organizations as the sole fount of medical wisdom, then the heterodox practitioners will continue to be considered as 'quacks' and 'untouchables'. For there is ample evidence to show that the orthodox medical power structure is just as capable of branding an orthodox practitioner who refuses to accept current medical thinking as a 'quack' and attempt to ostracize him. In this respect I am reminded of Sir Alexander Fleming, who said, 'Penicillin sat on a shelf for ten years while I was called a quack.'

In view of this attiude, before the new system of medicine can evolve, the people, the voting public, will have to make the practice of medicine a political issue, and demand that future representatives in London, Washington, Paris, Rome, and throughout the world, permit the alternative medical practitioner to have equal rights with his orthodox colleague. Once this is done, and not before, the door will be open to a total approach to medicine.

Now, if we assume this has been accomplished the second problem has to be analyzed, and this is three-sided.

On one side is the growing disenchantment of large sections of the population with orthodox medicine as it is felt it has become too depersonalized, and with the registered medical practitioner for being more interested in treating the disease than in helping the individual who is diseased.

The second side of the triangle is the increasing dislike and rejection of the over-usage and apparent abuse of drugs by members of the orthodoxy.

On the third side there is the allopathic preoccupation with disease rather than with health. This view was expressed by a registered medical practitioner from India when he was asked to compare the practice of medicine in his homeland with that of the West. His comment was, 'My only criticism of medicine in the West is that it is all based upon treating the sick, and not preventing the sickness.' In other words he highlighted the tremendous need we have for a personalized preventive medical programme to stop people from becoming ill and clogging up the present, and any future, medical system.

All this may appear to be obvious, and indeed there are signs that registered medical practitioners have begun to recognize the dilemma.

Proof that a change is underway can be seen in the courses now being offered in Britain for GPs by the Royal College of General Practitioners, which are meant to assist doctors in general practice to understand that people can be ill for a number of reasons, and that it is the task of the doctor not simply to treat the presenting symptom, but to try and locate the activating cause and remove that. Further confirmation of the wind of change was the decision made by the doctors in Ipswich to try and limit the number and size of drug prescriptions they were issuing. However, neither of these is enough. They are only permitting an old machine which has done admirable service in the past to continue to function a little longer before it finally expires of old age.

For it is well known that an old machine – and that is what medicine in its present form is – can only be adapted to meet future needs for a limited period of time; that is, until a new machine is built specifically to cope with the new conditions. And the new medical machine, so far not even on the drawing board as far as I have been able to ascertain, will be revolutionary by our present Western medical standards.

To meet the requirements of personalized preventive medicine, in all ante-natal clinics there will be nurses trained in the use of applied hypnosis to teach pregnant women how to relax into the hypnotic state and remain in it during childbirth so that they experience the least amount of discomfort while giving birth, and so that they also require the minimum amount of drugs or chemical anaesthesia in the process. This in itself is not revolutionary as there is at least one clinic in London where this is now being done, but as hypnosis has been known for more than a hundred years and is still not used to its full extent, this concept will have to be become the norm instead of the exception.

In addition to the nurse-hypnotist, each ante-natal clinic will have one or two manipulative therapists, and I use the term to cover osteopaths, chiropractors, or the eclectic manipulative therapists now emerging in Britain, to ensure that there are no skeletal abnormalities which could prevent the future mother from allowing her baby an easier emergence from the womb.

And still keeping to birth, it is more than probable that the position in which pregnant women are placed to have their babies will be altered, because there is now evidence coming from the United States of America to show that the 'squatting position' favoured by women in the East is both superior and more natural than that currently employed.

Equally in post-natal clinics there will be manipulative therapists to examine babies and mothers within weeks of the birth, and to correct any misalignment of the bones which may have been caused by the trauma of birth.

We may also find there is a medical herbalist attached to these clinics in case the small child suffers a minor illness, because, as a spokesman for the National Institute of Medical Herbalists told me, 'No young child should be given any drug as its system is unable to cope with it adequately, neither is it necessary because we have found that infants respond to herbal preparations very quickly.'

Continuing the programme of preventive medicine, at every school, from the day a child starts its schooling and all the way through until it leaves a college or university, there will be regular examinations by manipulative therapists to correct minor skeletal deformities, thereby preventing the formation of more serious conditions that may develop when the students are older.

All factories above a certain size will be encouraged to have a manipulative therapist on the staff to treat those who find they are experiencing discomfort due to the pressure of the work they are doing. And here it should be noted that this strain does not solely apply to manual workers, for physical stress can also affect the white-collar worker and the typist in exactly the same way.

Once the orthodox medical dictatorship has been replaced by medical democracy every hospital will have on its staff, in addition to the present medical complement, herbal, homeopathic and naturopathic practitioners who will work together harmoniously for the benefit of the patients in their united care, rather than fighting and striving to prove that any one therapeutic system is superior to another. The sole criteria of the hospital's medical staff will be, 'Which remedy will do the patient the least harm, and yet be effective.'

An illustration will show how this will work.

If a patient is admitted to hospital with appendicitis, and it is found by the admitting practitioner to be of such urgency that immediate surgery is imperative, then the surgeon and operating

L

theatre staff will be alerted to perform an appendectomy. However, should the appendix not be on the point of immediate rupturing, the patient would be referred to the homeopathic practitioner as the homeopaths have had remarkable results in treating cases of appendicitis without surgical intervention. Alternatively the patient would be passed to an acupuncturist, because there is evidence from medical centres in both China and Europe showing how the acupuncturist with his needles has been able to bring about a remission without resorting to surgery.[1]

Nor is this type of co-operation a pipe-dream. In China many hospitals have traditional medical practitioners, with herbalists and acupuncturists working alongside their allopathic colleagues without any competing for supremacy.

In the realm of general medical practice each branch of medicine will have its own Medical Association, none being subservient to the other, for if that happens, as it did in the United States with the osteopaths, the other Associaions would be quickly swallowed up. This will permit the individual to decide which practitioner he or she wants, and what type of medical approach is felt will suit the individual best.

And again in the field of general practice the various practitioners will be encouraged to obtain for their patients that form of treatment which they feel would be in the best interests of those needing care and attention. To accomplish this, instead of a proliferation of group medical practices that cause resentment among patients, there will be medical centres where practitioners of differing disciplines will have their offices. This will allow each GP to keep his or her own patients, while permitting them to refer an individual patient to a colleague in the same building.

An example of how this would work would be typified by a gentleman suffering from insomnia going to see an allopathic practitioner. The GP might prescribe a fourteen-day course of sleeping pills only to find that at the end of the course of treatment the condition had not improved, and that obviously a more prolonged therapeutic process was necessary. He could then decide that it was preferable for his patient to have a non-toxic course of treatment, and accordingly suggest that Mr Blank see a herbal or homeopathic colleague in the same building, who would make up a prescription to suit the individual's needs. But at all times the allopathic GP who was initially consulted would remain the patient's practitioner.

Of course the human medicine of the future would require the heterodox and orthodox practitioners to alter their attitudes, and lose some of their bigotry. There may be resentment in the beginning, but the answer to any such small-mindedness would be the words of the father of medicine, Hippocrates, who said on this subject: 'Nothing should be omitted in an art which interests the whole world, and which may be beneficial to suffering humanity and which does not risk human life or comfort.'

Notes

Chapter 1
1 Issue dated 10 February 1973.
2 *Pulse*, 3 March 1973.
3 'Learning to See Your Patients as People', *Pulse*, 3 February 1973.
4 For details of the hypno-diagnostic procedure see Chapter 7, *Hypnotism: Its Power and Practice* by Peter Blythe (Arthur Barker, London, 1971).
5 Issue dated 3 April 1973.
6 See the article 'Inquiry will only make things worse' by Dr Hertzel Creditor, *Pulse*, 3 February 1973.

Chapter 2
1 *General Practitioner* dated 18 April 1969.
2 *General Practitioner* dated 18 April 1969.
3 Issue dated 1 May 1972.
4 For confirmation see page 35 of *Fringe Medicine* by Brian Inglis (Faber and Faber, London, 1964).
5 Full details of this are to be found in 'Cell Therapy – Medicine of the Future', a three-part series of articles by Peter Stephan in the monthly magazine *Forum* (Vol. 4, Nos. 9–11), 2 Bramber Road, London.

Chapter 3
1 Issue dated May/June 1968.
2 Issue dated May/ June 1968.

Chapter 4

1 Details of the Hoxsey treatment for cancer and of what happened to it are fully recorded in the following chapter.
2 *British Herbal Pharmacopoeia* (British Herbal Medicine Association, London, 1972).
3 Published by Thorsons Publishers Ltd, London, 1968.
4 The letter was signed by A. Orbell, and reprinted in 'Fitness and Health from Herbs', dated October 1959.

Chapter 5

1 Published by the Kelley Research Foundation, Grapevine, Texas, 1969.
2 This was the earlier title of the booklet I had read; see 1 above.
3 Quoted from *The Defender* magazine, Witchita, Kansas, September 1952.
4 *Ibid*, December 1955.
5 See *Stress Disease: The Growing Plague*, Peter Blythe (Arthur Barker, London, 1973).
6 Published by the Arlin J. Brown Information Center, PO Box 251, Fort Belvoir, Virginia, 22060, USA.

Chapter 6

1 The Hoxsey Clinic has since been forced to close its doors, and it has to be remembered that this report was published in 1954.
2 The italics were in the original document.
3 The names of the doctors signing the document were: S. Edgar Bond, MD; Willard G. Palmer, MD; Hans Kalm, MD; A. C. Timbs, MD; Frederick H. Thurston, MD, DO; E. E. Loffler, MD; H. B. Mueller, MD; R. C. Bowie, MD; Benjamin F. Bowers, MD; Roy O. Yeatts, MD.
4 Extract from the report quoted earlier in this chapter.
5 Pages 5690–3.
6 What FitzGerald referred to was the allegation that Dr Andrew C. Ivy, a prominent medical man, Vice-President of the University of Illinois School of Medicine and a member of the Board of Directors of the American Cancer Society, became aware of Krebiozen, and

carried out a study of the effects of Krebiozen on cancer. He was impressed with the results and said so. After that he was approached by a leading member of the AMA who, on behalf of two Chicago businessmen, offered Dr Ivy $2,500,000 for exclusive distribution of Krebiozen. When Dr Ivy refused the offer he became a victim of a far-reaching conspiracy which included being called before the Board of Grievances of the Chicago Medical Society and charged with using a worthless drug for cancer.

7 Published by Hodder and Stoughton, London, 1973.

8 Issue dated 12 May 1972, under the heading 'Support for "Quacks" to Practise'.

Chapter 7

1 For full details of this conversation see the chapter 'Pills, Patients and People' in *Stress Disease: The Growing Plague*, Peter Blythe (Arthur Barker, London, 1973).

2 Published, London, 1958, and quoted in *Fringe Medicine*, Brian Inglis (Faber and Faber, London, 1964).

3 True Health Publishing Co, London, pages 75–6.

4 Full details are published in *Christian Samuel Hahnemann*, Rosa Waugh Hobhouse (the C. W. Daniel Co, Ltd. Ashingdon, Rochford, Essex, 1961).

5 'Homeopathy: A Case for Suitable Treatment' by Maggie Brittain, an article appearing in the *Lancashire Evening Post*, dated 13 October 1972.

6 'A Very Little of What You Fancy', *General Practitioner* dated 16 October 1970.

7 The Bach homeopathic remedies are regarded by the orthodoxy as less therapeutic than the regular homeopathic drugs because they come from the flowers of the field, and the tinctures are made by allowing the flower or herb to be exposed to the sun while lying in a small amount of distilled water.

To ease the minds of those involved in greyhound racing, the 'rescue' remedy is not a drug, nor could it normally affect the dog's racing performance in the same way as stimulants which are occasionally, and illegally, given.

8 An article appearing in *Homeopathic World,* Vol 47, by Dr J. R. P. Lambert.
9 Issue dated 24 February 1970.

Chapter 8

1 Virchow's italics.
2 Published by Boericke and Tafel, Philadephia, USA, 1911.
3 Peter Davies, London, 1970.
4 Gollancz, London, 1969; Corgi paperback edition January 1974.
5 *The Mating Game,* page 125.
6 Issue dated February 1971.
7 Reported in the *News of the World,* 29 April 1973.
8 Issue dated July 1963.
9 Published by the Hyppokrates Verlag, Stuttgart, Germany, 1955, and reviewed by the famous British osteopath, Mr Leslie Korth, DO, MRO, in *Fitness and Health Through Herbs,* May 1963.
10 Issue dated 28 April 1973.
11 *Everybody's Guide to Nature Cure* by Harry Benjamin (Health for All Publishing Co, London, 1961 edition, pages 79–80).
12 *Fitness and Health Through Herbs,* July 1963.

Chapter 9

1 Owing to the limited space available, this must be a generalization. There are some registered practitioners who have specialized in having a completely manipulative practice, and there is also a British Association of Manipulative Medicine, which conducts short courses for registered practitioners.
2 See *A Therapy for Anxiety Tension Reactions* by Drs Haugen, Dixon and Dickel (The Macmillan Company, New York, 1963).
3 Here the work of the neo-Reichian bio-energeticists at the Institute of Bio-energetics in New York City and others are referred to.

Chapter 10

1 Portland Printing House Company, 1910.
2 Quoted in 'Excerpt from Brief to Royal Commission on Health Services – 1962' (Canada), by D. C. Sutherland, DC.

3 Quoted from *Chiropractic: A Modern Way to Health* by Dr Julius Dintenfass, DC (Pyramid Books, New York, 1966, pp. 21–22).
4 One of the acknowledged Colleges is the Anglo-European in Bournemouth, England, and the Danish Pro-Chiropractic Association annually contributes £2,000 to it.
5 Issue dated August 1972.
6 'Anxiety-Depression and Cervical Joint Trauma' by Dr John Ebbetts, issue dated 26 January 1973.
7 Issue dated February 1961.

Chapter 11
1 See *Hypnotism: Its Power and Practice*, Chapter 7.
2 For further details see Chapter 4, The Rhythms of the Body, in *Wilhelm Reich: The Evolution of his Work* by David Boadella (Vision Press, London, 1973).
3 *Fundamentals of Psychoanalytic Technique* (Wiley, New York, 1954).
4 *Betrayal of the Body* by Dr Alexander Lowen (Collier Books, New York, 1967).
5 *The Primal Scream* by Dr Arthur Janov (Dell Publishing Co, New York, 1970).
6 Since this case, the routine I use has been further refined and made more accurate. All I have done above is to relate how I discovered that hypnosis is ready to grow up and develop into a therapy with a far wider application than previously considered.

Chapter 12
1 The Chinese Medical Journal, dated February 1960, in a piece entitled 'Acupuncture in the Treatment of Acute Appendicitis', reported that out of 116 cases treated with acupuncture 92.5 per cent recovered within six days without requiring surgery.

Bibliography

Béchamp, Prof. A., *The Blood and Its Third Anatomical Element* (Boericke and Tafel, Philadephia, USA, 1911)

Benjamin, Harry, *Everybody's Guide to Nature Cure* (Health for All Publishing Co., London, 1961 edition)

Blythe, Peter, *Hypnotism: Its Power and Practice* (Arthur Barker, London, 1971)

Blythe, Peter, *Stress Disease: The Growing Plague* (Arthur Barker, London, 1973)

Boadella, David, *Wilhelm Reich: The Evolution of his Work* (Vision Press, London, 1973)

Braaty, Trygve, *Fundamentals of Psychoanalytic Technique* (Wiley, New York, 1954)

British Herbal Medicine Association, *British Herbal Pharmacopoeia* (London, 1971)

Brown, Arlin J, *March of Truth on Cancer* (PO Box 251, Fort Belvoir, Virginia, USA)

Dintenfass, Dr Julius, *Chiropractic: A Modern Way to Health* (Pyramid Books, New York, 1966)

Haugen, Dr G. B., Dixon, Dr H. H., and Dickel, Dr H. A., *A Therapy for Anxiety Tension Reactions* (The Macmillan Company, New York, 1963)

Hewlett-Parsons, J., *Herbs, Health and Healing* (Thorsons, London, 1968)

Hobhouse, Rosa Waugh, *Christian Samuel Hahnemann* (C. W. Daniel, Ashingdon, Rochford, Esssex, 1961)

Inglis, Brian, *Fringe Medicine* (Faber and Faber, London, 1964)

Johns, June, *The Mating Game* (Peter Davies, London, 1970)

Johns, June, *Zoo Without Bars* (Gollancz, London, 1969)

Janov, Dr Arthur, *The Primal Scream* (Dell Publishing Company, New York, 1970)

Kelley, Dr William D., *New Hope for Cancer Victims* (The Kelley Foundation, Grapevine, Texas, 1969)

Lowen, Dr Alexander, *Betrayal of the Body* (Collier Books, New York, 1967)

Palmer, D. D., *The Science and Art and Philosophy of Chiropractic* (Portland Printing House Company, 1910)

Roueché, Berton, *The Incurable Wound* (London, 1958)

Scott, Cyril, *Medicine – Rational and Irrational* (True Health Publishing Co, London)

Thomas, Gordon, *Issels: The Biography of a Doctor* (Hodder and Stoughton, London, 1973)

Tienes, Dr George A., *Der Baunscheidtismus* (Hyppokrates Verlag, Stuttgart, Germany, 1955)

Index